Diagnosis Of Dental Caries ~ Old And The New

OrangeBooks Publication

Smriti Nagar, Bhilai, Chhattisgarh - 490020

Website: **www.orangebooks.in**

First Edition, 2022

ISBN: 978-93-92878-57-2

The opinions/ contents expressed in this book are solely of the authors and do not represent the opinions/ standings/ thoughts of OrangeBooks or the Editors .

Printed in India

DIAGNOSIS OF DENTAL CARIES ~ OLD AND THE NEW

Dr Sana Farooq

MDS Deparment Of Pedodontics
And Preventive Dentistry

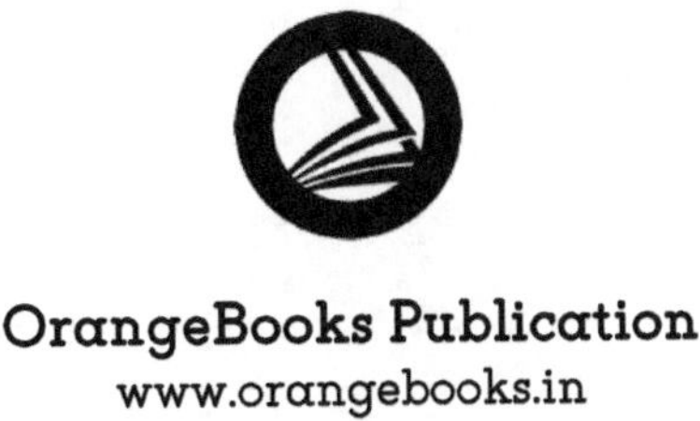

OrangeBooks Publication
www.orangebooks.in

Table Of Contents

Introduction

Dental caries which is prevelant worldwide may be defined as a dynamic disease process, in which early lesions undergo many demineralization and remineralization cycles before being expressed clinically.[1] It is a complex disease, defined as a progressive, irreversible, microbial disease affecting the hard parts of the tooth exposed to the oral environment, characterized by demineralization of inorganic constituents and destruction of the organic constituents thereby leading to a cavity formation. As long as the dynamic equilibrium between the mineral content of the tooth-oral fluid and the microbial content of the biofilm are maintained, the entire sequence remains within the boundary of a physiological process, where loss and gain are equalized.[2]

The change of dental caries from a physiological process to pathology is a continuous process and is affected by numerous variables and also there is a lack of a specific boundary line between health and disease. The progression of non cavitated lesions seems to be slower, allowing preventive strategies to be implemented when the lesions have the greatest opportunity to arrest.[3] So , early and accurate detection and diagnosis of dental caries are an important component of the overall management of dental patient. It is imperative that the diagnostic methods with suitable level of sensitivity and specificity are used in conjunction to obtain a valid diagnosis. [2]

Early **recognition of the initiation** and **early detection of caries** should be the primary concern rather than the search for cavities for a dentist and it reduces irreversible loss of tooth structure, the subsequent treatment costs and time needed for restoration of the teeth.[4]

Dental caries affects 60-90% of school children and almost 100% of adult population is affected and progression of **non-cavitated lesions** seems to be slower allowing preventive strategies to be implemented when the lesions have the greatest opportunity to arrest.

Ideally, a diagnostic tool should detect dental caries at its earliest stage possible, provide valid prospective caries risk assessments for different age groups and determine present caries activity and monitor lesions behaviour over time.[5]

The ideal requisites of Diagnosing Aid is that it is accuracte, reliable, precise/simple, easy to apply, useful for all surfaces of teeth, identify caries adjacent to restoration , should be objective, sensitive , specific , results should be reproducible, valid and used for quantitative analysis.[6] It should be easy to apply, be useful for all surfaces of the tooth including caries adjacent to restorations, should assess the activity of the lesion, and should be sensitive, allowing lesions to be detected at early stages.

Diagnostic methods become the science behind the creation of diagnosis and a clinician requires knowledge, ability, and skill to apply the right diagnostic method and to interpret them. Earlier Visual examination using mouth mirrors, probes, and conventional radiography were the diagnostic methods used to diagnose caries. Literature indicate that the use of probe has been limited in caries detection and is also known to disrupt remineralization.

Traditional Methods combined with more sensitive methods may improve the caries diagnosis help in clinician in monitoring non-operative treatments. The original maxim of "extension for prevention" has been replaced by a minimal intervention approach.

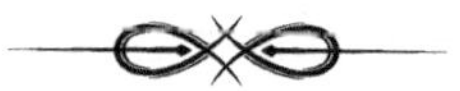

An International Consensus Workshop On Caries Clinical Trials (Icw-Cct) Concluded That : 7

- Lesion detection implies an objective method of determining whether or not the disease is present, lesion assessment which aims to characterize it once it has been detected and caries diagnosis which implies a human professional summation of all available data.

- Visual diagnosis is the standard of caries diagnosis and the use of additional methods should be explored further.

- Bitewing radiography adds information to the diagnosis and in future clinical trials, recording only cavitated lesions as an outcome is needed

- Caries measurement methods should accurately capture any signs of the manifestations of the caries process at any given point in time, be able to monitor different levels of de/remineralisation and differentiate product effects in terms of lesion initiation and determine progression, arrest or regression of lesion behaviour .

Preventive strategies have not been utilized efficiently by the dental professional because of failure to observe successful outcomes, financial pressures and the inability to detect lesions at an early stage sufficient for effective prevention and operative care has been central management strategy for caries control in general practice which has negatively impacted on caries epidemiology, clinical outcomes, and patients' quality of life.

Diagnosis is "the art or act of identifying a disease from its signs and symptoms" and caries detection is the signs and symptoms identified. These two terms have been confusing in past and used interchangeably.

Lesion detection implies to an objective method of determining whether or not disease is present; whereas lesion assessment aims to characterise or monitor a lesion, once it has been detected, and caries diagnosis implies a human, professional, summation of all available data.

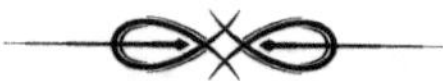

Caries Risk Assessment

It is one of the cornerstones in caries management and should be carried out and documented in the patient's chart either for treatment planning or as a didactic patient modification aid.

Caries risk assessment (CRA) is the process of establishing the probability of an individual patient, or groups of children, developing carious lesions over a certain time period or the likelihood that there will be a change in size or activity of lesions already present .[8]

Studies have helped in correctly identifying the individuals at risk for caries, which is the determining characteristic of an ideal **CRA** system and labelling a child as moderate risk, high risk and low risk group.

Factors	High risk	Moderate risk	Low Risk
Risk factors, social/biological			
Mother/primary caregiver has active dental caries	Yes		
Parent/caregiver has life-time of poverty, low health literacy	Yes		
Child has frequent exposure (>3 times/day) between-meal sugar-containing snacks or beverages per day	Yes		
Child uses bottle or non-spill cup containing natural or added sugar frequently, between meals and/or at bedtime	Yes		

	High risk	Moderate risk	Low risk
Child is a recent immigrant		Yes	
Child has special health care needs		Yes	
Protective factors			
Child receives optimally-fluoridated drinking water or fluoride supplements			Yes
Child has teeth brushed daily with fluoridated toothpaste			Yes
Child receives topical fluoride from health professional			Yes
Child has dental home/regular dental care			Yes
Clinical findings			
Child has non-cavitated (incipient/white spot) caries or enamel defects	Yes		
Child has visible cavities or fillings or missing teeth due to caries	Yes		
Child has visible plaque on teeth	Yes		

Table 1: Caries-risk Assessment Form for 0-5 Years Old

Factors	High risk	Moderate risk	Low risk
Risk factors, social/biological			
Patient has life-time of poverty, low health literacy	Yes		
Patient has frequent exposure (>3 times/day) between-meal sugar-	Yes		

containing snacks or beverages per day			
Child is a recent immigrant		Yes	
Patient has special health care needs		Yes	
Protective factors Patient receives optimally-fluoridated drinking water			Yes
Patient brushes teeth daily with fluoridated toothpaste			Yes
Patient receives topical fluoride from health professional			Yes
Patient has dental home/regular dental care			Yes
Clinical findings Patient has al interproximal caries lesions	Yes		
Patient has active non-cavitated (white spot) caries lesions or enamel defects	Yes		
Patient has low salivary flow	Yes		
Patient has defective restorations		Yes	
Patient wears an intraoral appliance		Yes	

Table 2: Caries-Risk Assessment Form For Greater Than 6 Years

ADA American Dental Association®
America's leading advocate for oral health

Caries Risk Assessment Form (Age >6)

Patient Name:

Birth Date:

Date:

Age:

Initials:

		Low Risk	Moderate Risk	High Risk
Contributing Conditions		**Check or Circle the conditions that apply**		
I.	Fluoride Exposure (through drinking water, supplements, professional applications, toothpaste)	☐ Yes	☐ No	
II.	Sugary Foods or Drinks (including juice, carbonated or non-carbonated soft drinks, energy drinks, medicinal syrups)	Primarily at mealtimes ☐		Frequent or prolonged between meal exposures/day ☐
III.	Caries Experience of Mother, Caregiver and/or other Siblings (for patients ages 6-14)	No carious lesions in last 24 months ☐	Carious lesions in last 7-23 months ☐	Carious lesions in last 6 months ☐
IV.	Dental Home: established patient of record, receiving regular dental care in a dental office	☐ Yes	☐ No	
General Health Conditions		**Check or Circle the conditions that apply**		
I.	Special Health Care Needs (developmental, physical, medical or mental disabilities that prevent or limit performance of adequate oral health care by themselves or caregivers)	☐ No	Yes (over age 14) ☐	Yes (ages 6-14) ☐
II.	Chemo/Radiation Therapy	☐ No		☐ Yes
III.	Eating Disorders	☐ No	☐ Yes	
IV.	Medications that Reduce Salivary Flow	☐ No	☐ Yes	
V.	Drug/Alcohol Abuse	☐ No	☐ Yes	

	Clinical Conditions	**Check or Circle the conditions that apply**		
I.	Cavitated or Non-Cavitated (incipient) Carious Lesions or Restorations (visually or radiographically evident)	No new carious lesions or restorations in last 36 months ☐	1 or 2 new carious lesions or restorations in last 36 months ☐	3 or more carious lesions or restorations in last 36 months ☐
II.	Teeth Missing Due to Caries in past 36 months	☐ No		☐ Yes
III.	Visible Plaque	☐ No	☐ Yes	
IV.	Unusual Tooth Morphology that compromises oral hygiene	☐ No	☐ Yes	
V.	Interproximal Restorations - 1 or more	☐ No	☐ Yes	
VI.	Exposed Root Surfaces Present	☐ No	☐ Yes	
VII.	Restorations with Overhangs and/or Open Margins; Open Contacts with Food Impaction	☐ No	☐ Yes	
VIII.	Dental/Orthodontic Appliances (fixed or removable)	☐ No	☐ Yes	
IX.	Severe Dry Mouth (Xerostomia)	☐ No		☐ Yes

Overall assessment of dental caries risk: ☐ Low   ☐ Moderate   ☐ High

Patient Instructions:

Table 3: Aapd Caries Risk Assessment Tool (Cat)

Risk Factors To Consider	High Risk	Moderate Risk	Low Risk
Part I – History			
Child has SPHCN, especially any that impact motor coordination or co-operation	Yes		No
Child has condition that impairs saliva (dry mouth)	Yes		No
Child' s use of dental home (frequency of routine visits)	None	Irregular	Regular
Child has decay	Yes		No
Time lapsed since child's last cavity	<12 mnths	12-24 mnths	>24 mnths
Child has braces or wears orthodontic appliances	Yes		No
Risk Factors To Consider	**High Risk**	**Moderate Risk**	**Low Risk**
Child's parent and/or siblings have decay	Yes		No
Socioeconomic status of the child's parent	Low	Mid level	high
Daily b/w meals exposure to sugar/ cavity producing foods (includes on demand use of bottle/ sippy cup containing liquid other than water, consumption of juice,	>3	1-2	Meal time only

carbonated beverages, sports drinks, use of sweetened medications)			
Child's exposure to F	Doesnot use F tooth paste, drinking water is not F, not taking F supplements	Uses F tooth paste, usually does not drink Fwater & does not taking F supplements	Uses F tooth paste, drinks Fwater or takes F supplements
Time/day that child's teeth or gums are brushed	<1	1	2-3

Risk Factors To Consider	High Risk	Moderate Risk	Low Risk
Part II – Clinical Evaluation			
Visible plaque (white, sticky build up)	Present		Absent
Gingivitis (red, puffy gums)	Present		Absent
Areas of demineralisation (chalky, white spots on teeth)	>1	1	None
Enamel defects, deep P/F	Present		Absent
PART III – Supplemental Professional Assessment (optional)			
R/g enamel caries	Present		Absent
Level of MS or lactobacilli	High	Moderate	Low

Table 4: Difference Between High, Moderate And Low Caries Risk Group

Risk Category	Diagnostics	Interventions			Restorative
		Fluoride	Dietary Counseling	Sealants	
Low risk	– Recall every six to 12 months – Radiographs every 12 to 24 months	– Drink optimally fluoridated water – Twice daily brushing with fluoridated toothpaste	Yes	Yes	– Surveillance
Moderate risk	– Recall every six months – Radiographs every six to 12 months	– Drink optimally fluoridated water – Twice daily brushing with fluoridated toothpaste – Fluoride supplements – Professional topical treatment every six months	Yes	Yes	– Active surveillance of non-cavitated (white spot) caries lesions – Restore of cavitated or enlarging caries lesions
High risk	– Recall every three months – Radiographs every six months	– Drink optimally fluoridated water – Twice daily brushing with fluoridated toothpaste – Professional topical treatment every three months – Silver diamine fluoride on cavitated lesions	Yes	Yes	– Active surveillance of non-cavitated (white spot) caries lesions – Restore of cavitated or enlarging caries lesions

Table 5: Example Of A Caries Management Pathways For 0-5 Years Old

Risk Category	Diagnostics	Interventions			Restorative
		Fluoride	Dietary Counseling	Sealants	
Low risk	– Recall every six to 12 months – Radiographs every 12 to 24 months	– Drink optimally fluoridated water – Twice daily brushing with fluoridated toothpaste	Yes	Yes	– Surveillance
Moderate risk	– Recall every six months – Radiographs every six to 12 months	– Drink optimally fluoridated water – Twice daily brushing with fluoridated toothpaste – Fluoride supplements – Professional topical treatment every six months	Yes	Yes	– Active surveillance of non-cavitated (white spot) caries lesions – Restore of cavitated or enlarging caries lesions
High risk	– Recall every three months – Radiographs every six months	– Drink optimally fluoridated water – Brushing with 0.5 percent fluoride gel/paste – Professional topical treatment every three months – Silver diamine fluoride on cavitated lesions	Yes	Yes	– Active surveillance of non-cavitated (white spot) caries lesions – Restore of cavitated or enlarging caries lesions

Table 6: Example Of A Caries Management Pathways For ≥6 Years Old

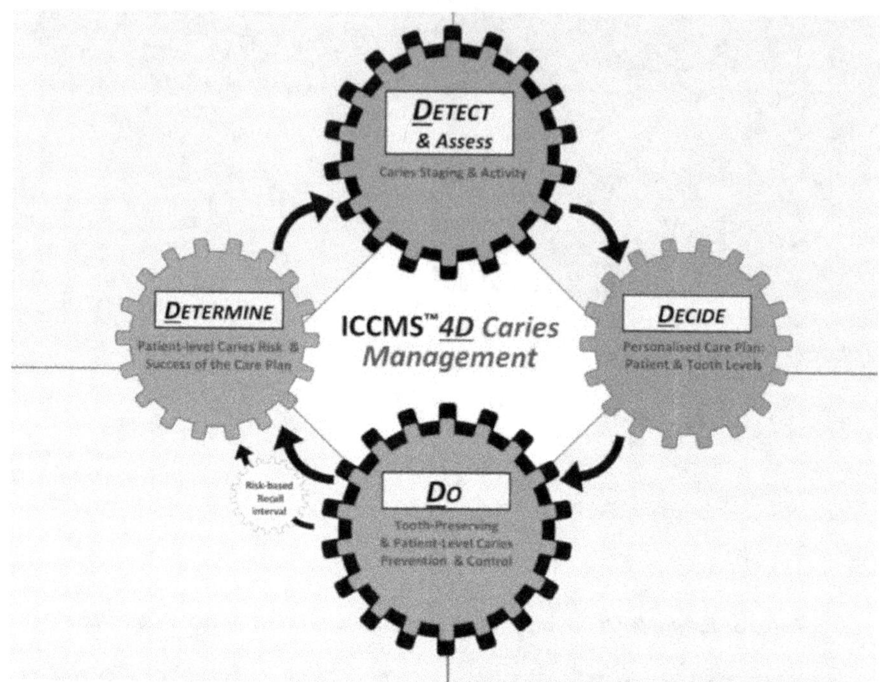

Figure 1: Caries outcomes focused model that aims to maintain health and preserve tooth structure using a personalized, risk-based management

Four well-known ones are CAMBRA, Cariogram, American Dental Association (ADA), and American Academy of Pediatric Dentistry (AAPD) CRAs. Both the Cariogram and the CAMBRA CRA methods are equally useful for identifying the future risk of dental caries.

Renata Nunes CABRAL , Leandro Augusto Hilgert, Soraya Coelho Leal conducted a study titled Caries risk assessment in schoolchildren - a form based on **Cariogram® software** with the aim of this study was to determine whether a newly developed Caries Risk Assessment (CRA) form based on the Cariogram® software could classify schoolchildren according to their caries risk and to evaluate relationships between caries risk and the variables in the form. Identifying caries risk factors is an important measure which contributes to best understanding of the cariogenic profile of the patient. The Cariogram® software provides this analysis, and protocols simplifying the method were suggested. 150 schoolchildren aged 5 to 7 years old were included in this survey. Caries prevalence was obtained according to International Caries Detection and

Assessment System (ICDAS) II. Information for filling in the form based on Cariogram® was collected clinically and from questionnaires sent to parents. Linear regression and a forward stepwise multiple regression model were applied to correlate the variables included in the form with the caries risk.[9]

Caries prevalence, in primary dentition, including enamel and dentine carious lesions was 98.6%, and 77.3% when only dentine lesions were considered. Eighty-six percent of the children were classified as at moderate caries risk. The forward stepwise multiple regression model result was significant ($R2=0.904$; $p<0.00001$), showing that the most significant factors influencing caries risk were caries experience, oral hygiene, frequency of food consumption, sugar consumption and fluoride sources.

The study concluded the use of the form based on the Cariogram®software enabled classification of the schoolchildren at low, moderate and high caries risk. Caries experience, oral hygiene, frequency of food consumption, sugar consumption and fluoride sources are the variables that were shown to be highly correlated with caries risk.

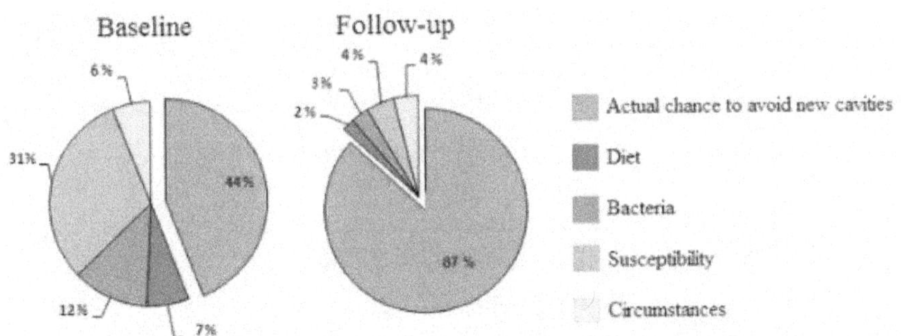

Figure 2: Cariogram Sectors At Baseline And Follow Up

Physical principle	Application in caries detection
X-rays	Digital subtraction radiography Digital image enhancement
Visible light	Fibre optic transillumination (FOTI) Quantitative light-induced fluorescence(QLF) Digital image fibre optictransillumination(DiFOTI)
Laser light	Laser fluorescence measurement (DiagnoDent)
Electrical current	Electrical conductance measurement (ECM) Electrical impedance measurement
Ultrasound	Ultrasonic caries detector

Table 7: Physical Principles Behind Caries Detection Instrument

S No	Diagnostic Principle	Advancements
01	Visual	MOUTH MIRROR ICDAS
02	Radiography	RVG Bitewing radiography Xeroradiography CBCT IOPAR Digital Subraction radiography TACT
03	Laser	Laser assisted DIFOTI Cariescan
04	Transillumination	FOTI DIFOTI Wavelength dependant FOTI
05	Fluorescence	QLF Soprolife Diagnodent

06	Electric Current	Electric conductance measurement
		Electric impedance measurement
07	Ultrasound	Ultrasound caries monitor

Table 8: Diagnostic Aids For Caries Used In Pediatric Dentistry

Diagnostic aids	Advantages	Disadvantages
Digital radiography	Instant and consistent image No dark room needed Eliminates hazards of fil development Capable of teletransmission	High cost Life expectancy of chip
Digital image enhancement	Contrast can be digitally enhanced	Time consuming
Digital subtraction radiography	Detects onset or progression of demineralization	Difficulty of image registration
Tuned aperture computed tomography	Detect small primary and secidary carious lesion	Technique sensitive
VISIBLE LIGHT		
OPTICAL CARIES MONITOR	No hazards Lesion not diagnoised by radiographs can be diagnosed	Inter and intraobserver variations Low sensitivity
Digital imaging fiber optic transillumination	Detects initial areas of demineralization	

	Inspects integrity of teeth Detects cracks, tooth fractures and wears No harmful radiation Use safe white light Images all coronal surfaces including	

Table 9: Advantages and disadvantages of advanced diagnostic methods for early detection of caries

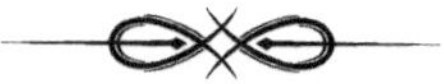

Pathophysiology, Histopathology, Evaluation And Differential Diagnosis

Pathophysiology

The initial source of *S. mutans* in infants is usually from the mother, most likely via free-floating organisms in saliva. Most studies indicate that infants become colonized before the eruption of the first primary tooth. Infants with mothers who have high levels of *S. mutans* have a greater risk of acquiring *S. mutans* earlier than children whose mothers have low levels. The horizontal transmission also occurs.

Dental biofilm is an aggregate of microorganisms in which cells adhere to each other and to a surface. This aggregate of cells is encapsulated in a self-produced organic matrix of polysaccharides, proteins, and DNA. The significance of the dental biofilm is that it enhances the cariogenicity of acid-producing bacteria by protecting these bacteria from host defense.

The oral cavity is a unique microbiological habitat; it allows for distinct ecological niches. There are shedding surfaces (soft tissue), non-shedding surfaces (teeth), saliva, and others; each of these is a separate ecological niche. Colonization of these locations is dependent upon the characteristics of the specific organism and microbiological niche. Saliva is a medium for free-floating or planktonic bacteria.[10]

Histopathology:

A carious tissue consists of four different zones histologically, among which three zones are visible clinically. The outer layer consists of the necrotic zone and contaminated zone containing microbial biofilm, which can be appreciated clinically as soft mineralized tissue of the tooth. This necrotic zone has a very high microbial load. The next zone is the zone of demineralization characterized by very few microorganisms, minimal nutrients, and an anaerobic atmosphere. This zone can be correlated clinically as leathery dentine. Finally, the innermost zone located near the pulp is the translucent zone of firm softer dentine. Demineralization and the absence of microorganisms characterize this zone because microbial flora cannot penetrate till this depth.

History /Physical

History: The patients with dental caries present with various symptoms depending on the extent of carious involvement. For the initial lesion, which represents a white spot on the tooth surface, the patients complain of a surface discoloration on the particular teeth. Some of the patients present with food lodged in the area affected, which may be due to cavitation of the tooth. If caries have progressed close to the pulp, the patients may complain of pain. The severity of pain may differ based on the stage of involvement, extent, loss of hard structure, and host reparative response.

Physical: The most common method used for the physical evaluation of dental caries is the use of a dental mouth mirror and explorer. If there is a presence of a "catch" on the tooth surface along with the loss of some tooth structure, caries may be suspected.

Evaluation:

Evaluation of dental caries involves the use of various techniques like visual-tactile method, radiographs, chemical methods that include the use of caries detecting dyes, and most recent techniques like the use of fiberoptic illumination (FOTI), digital fiberoptic illumination (DIFOTI), and electric caries monitor. The most common and easiest method is the conventional visual-tactile method in which the examiner uses a dental mouth mirror and straight explorer along with the clinical judgment. To detect caries radiographically, several radiographic techniques are effective, such as intraoral periapical radiograph, bitewing radiograph for occluso-proximal caries, and radiovisiography, based on the density of sound and carious hard tooth structure. Digital techniques include fiber-optic transillumination (FOTI), digital imaging fiber-optic transillumination (DIFOTI), which works on the principle of optical transillumination. Chemical methods include the use of various dyes that are used to stain the collagenous part of the carious tooth structure, thereby delineating affected and non affected tooth structure. The most recent method is a caries meter, based on the principle that as the carious process progress, there is an increase in pore volume and porosity at the microstructure level, which increases the electrical conductance.

Differential Diagnosis of dental caries includes:

- Dental fluorosis

- Developmental disorders encompassing: hypomineralization and hypoplasia of the tooth, white spot lesion or periapical pathology, and pigmented lesion of the tooth.

The Concept Of Caries Diagnosis

The proper management of dental caries in clinical practice requires an accurate diagnosis. So before deciding on a treatment plan which may include a range of clinical techniques, the characteristics of the manifestations of the caries disease of the individual child must be assessed.

Dental caries is the localized destruction of susceptible dental hard tissues by acidic by products from bacterial fermentation of dietary carbohydrates where disease process is initiated within the bacterial biofilm (dental plaque) that covers the tooth surface. The process is dynamic and numerous episodes of loss and gain of mineral (demineralization and remineralization) take place on the enamel surface. If demineralization prevails over remineralization the result will be permanent and irreversible loss of mineral, cavity formation, and complete continuous destruction of hard tissues .

The signs and symptoms of this disease starts from the smallest subsurface loss of minerals to severe destruction of the tooth. In clinical practice, the signs and symptoms of the carious demineralization describe the disease once it is detectable by visual–tactile examination possibly combined with other diagnostic methods such as radiography. [11]

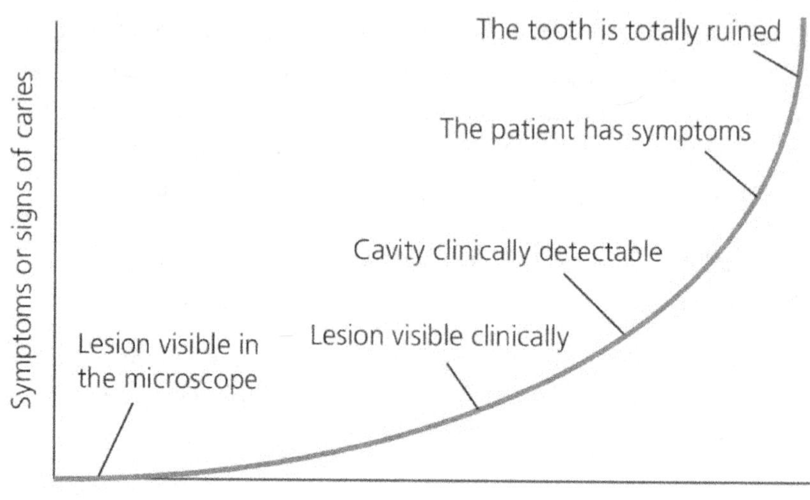

Figure 3: Graph Depicting Symptoms Or Signs Of Caries Over Time

Occlusal pits and fissures		Smooth surfaces	
Inactive	**Active**	**Inactive**	**Active**
Persistence of the lesions over years/decades	Detection within some years after tooth eruption	Persistence of the lesions over years/decades	Detection within some years after tooth eruption
No plaque coverage	Plaque coverage	No plaque coverage	Plaque coverage
Glossy, shiny appearance of the enamel surface after air-drying	Matt/frosty/rough appearance of the enamel surface after air-drying	Glossy, shiny appearance of the enamel surface after air-drying	Matt/frosty/rough appearance of the enamel surface after air-drying
No pathological enlargements	Microcavities	Lesions located in distance to the gingiva	White spots near the gingiva margin
Brown discoloration in enamel	White(-brown) discoloration in enamel	Brown discoloration in enamel	White(-brown) discoloration in enamel
Hard, dry, discolored dentine	Soft, wet, (un)discolored dentine	Hard, dry, discolored dentine	Soft, wet, (un)discolored dentine

Table 10: Clinical Indicators Of Inactive And Active Caries Lesions On Occlusal And Smooth Surfaces.

The various diagnostic aids can be categorized as:

- Routine diagnostic aids
- Specialized diagnostic aids
- Advanced diagnostic aids.

Routine diagnostic aids: The clinical intraoral examination is performed systematically in a clean, dry, well-illuminated mouth using the mouth mirror, explorer and periodontal probe.

Specialized diagnostic aids: These are used for the diagnosis of specific dental problems like detection of dental caries, pulpal diseases and orthodontic problems.

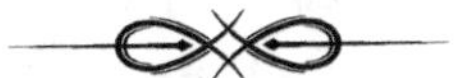

Diagnosis Of Dental Caries

Dental caries is a chronic disease that involves destruction of tooth structure, which can lead to loss of masticatory function and unesthetic appearance of affected enamel. The boundaries of caries diagnosis and caries interventions are changing. Dentists currently use visual, tactile and radiographic information to detect relatively advanced changes in the dental hard tissues. Diagnosis of dental caries is often regarded as synonymous with the detection of clinical signs of tissue damage caused by the disease, i.e carious lesions and cavities.

Methods of Clinical Diagnosis of Dental Caries

Dental caries is a dynamic process and accurate diagnosis of the very incipient stages of a carious lesion can result in its reversal by the use of proper intervention methods:

- **Clinical Method (Visual-Tactile Method):** GV Black in1924 suggested the use of a sharp explorer to examine dental caries and the tooth surface was counted as decayed if slight pull was required to remove the explorer from the tooth surface. The same suggestion was given by Simon in 1956, Gillmore in 1982, and Marzouk and Sturdevant in 1985. Today it has been proved that the explorer point may fracture the demineralized enamel leading to cavitations. Use of a mirror and blunt probe is the most common method of diagnosing tooth decay. A sharp probe can break the intact tooth surface and one of the enamel lesions causing a cavity. [12]

- **Radiographic Methods:** Radiographs can be classified into the conventional and advanced techniques. Though, conventional radiographs like bitewing and intraoral periapical radiograph are most frequently used for the detection of caries, they may cause overlapping of teeth due to faulty angulations and may also miss the initial lesion. During the primary dentition, the occlusal surface is most susceptible to caries attack, but with the eruption of first permanent molars the incidence of proximal lesions greatly increases. In such situation, bitewing radiographs are absolutely required to detect proximal lesions in primary molars.

The Advanced radiographic techniques include digital radiography and xeroradiography. Digital radiography is a digital, filmless technique for intraoral radiography, utilizes very little of the radiation to which the patient has been exposed and avoids the need for developing films. Xeroradiography has the advantages of producing less radiation and edge enhancement along with its wide latitude of exposure.

Figure 4: RVG

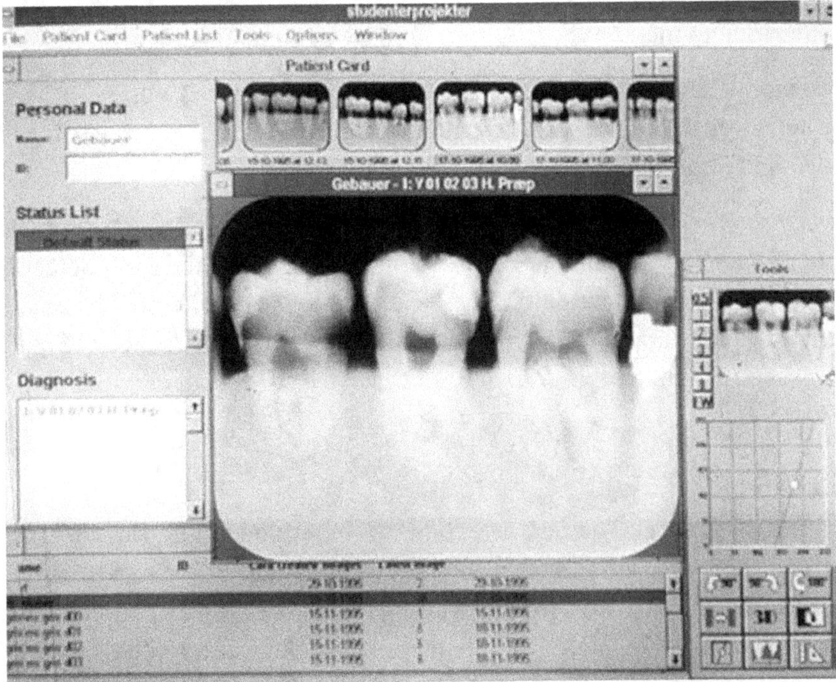

Tooth separation :

In this method orthodontic modules or bands can be used to achieve slow separation and by separating the teeth one can visualize the proximal and approximal surfaces.

Visual Inspection

The most common diagnosis methods implemented by dentists to make an accurate assessment is visual inspection and for that the teeth should be clean, dry and examined under a light source. Visually changes in tooth structure like enamel dissolution, white spot lesions, discolouration, surface roughness and presence of cavitation are assessed. So illuminating carious tissues tend to scatter the light and make enamel look whiter and opaque due to increased porosity caused by demineralization.

Demineralization of dentin leads to a shadow which is observed under the intact enamel and with dental caries progression the surface breaks down and a cavitation is formed .

International Consensus Workshop on Caries Clinical Trials which was held in Scotland in 2002 had stressed on importance of the early detection of caries which was emphasized and the idea of development of *International Caries Detection and Assessment System (ICDAS)* was proposed. In 2005, the *ICDAS* criteria was revised and published as *ICDAS II* .[13]

ICDAS :

Currently available caries detection to practitioners is *International Caries Detection and Assessment System (ICDAS)* system that was developed in 2001 by an international group of researchers. It was proposed as a strategy to integrate the modern detection systems into one standard system .

The ICDAS incorporate concepts from the research conducted by **Ekstrand** *et al.* **Fyffe** *et al.* and other caries detection systems described in the systematic review conducted by **Ismail** (2004) . The ICDAS is the subdivision of stages of the continuum of dental caries into a variable number of discrete and predictable categories based upon the histological extent of the lesion within the tooth . It identifies caries lesions on the basis of their clinical visual appearance where visual aided ball-ended explorer should be carried out on clean and dry teeth .

The assessment of lesion activity is also very important when using ICDAS where Lesion activity assessment will help on the treatment decisions, particularly when preventive options should be implemented . ICDAS has shown to be an accurate and reproducible method to detect early lesions and also to detect changes in longitudinal follow-up .

Nyvad criteria	ICDAS criteria
Lesion severity and activity are determined as one score.	Severity score and activity assessment are provided as two separate scores.
These criteria are applied to plaque-covered teeth.	These criteria are initiated on cleaned teeth.
A sharp probe is used.	The use of a ball-ended probe is recommended.

Table 11: Difference Between Nygard And Icdas Scoring

ICDAS scores

Score	Criteria
0	Sound
1	First Visual Change in enamel
2	Distinct Visual Change in enamel
3	Localized enamel breakdown
4	Underlying dentine shadow
5	Distinct cavity with visible dentine
6	Extensive cavity with visible dentine

Table 12: Scoring Criteria Of Icdas

ICDAS Lay Terms	Sound	Early Stage Decay		Established Decay		Severe Decay	
ICDAS Dental Terms	Sound	First visual change in enamel	Distinct visual change in enamel	Localised enamel breakdown	Underlying dentine shadow	Distinct cavity with visible dentine	Extensive cavity within visible dentine
ICDAS Detection	0	1	2	3	4	5	6
ICDAS Activity				ICDAS Activity +/-			

Table 13: ICDAS Detection Terms

ICDAS gives reliable and accurate results in identification of early caries lesions and changes taking place in the long term .The basic codes are given as follows;

0. Sound tooth surface,

1. First visual change in enamel,

2. Distinct visual change in enamel,

3. Localized enamel breakdown due to caries with no visible dentin,

4. Underlying dark shadow from dentin (with or without enamel breakdown),

5. Distinct cavity with visible dentin,

6. Extensive distinct cavity with visible dentin.

Codes of description :
Pit and Fissure Caries[9]

Code 0: Sound Tooth Surface

There should be no evidence of caries (either no or questionable) change in enamel translucency after prolonged air drying (suggested drying time 5 seconds). Surfaces with developmental defects, such as enamel hypoplasias, fluorosis, tooth wear (attrition, abrasion and erosion), and extrinsic or intrinsic stains will be recorded as sound. The examiner should also score as sound a surface with multiple stained fissures if such a condition is seen in other pits and fissures, a condition which is consistent with noncarious habits (e.g. frequent tea drinking).[14]

Code 1: First Visual Change in Enamel

When seen wet there is no evidence of any change in color attributable to carious activity, but after prolonged air drying, a carious opacity or discoloration (white or brown lesion) is visible that is not consistent with the clinical appearance of sound enamel or when there is a change of color due to caries which is not consistent with the clinical appearance of sound enamel and is limited to the confines of the pit and fissure area (whether seen wet or dry). The appearance of these carious areas is not consistent with that of stained pits and fissures as defined in code 0.

Code 2: Distinct Visual Change in Enamel

The tooth must be viewed wet. When wet there is a carious opacity (white spot lesion) and/or brown carious discoloration which is wider than the natural fissure/fossa that is not consistent with the clinical appearance of sound enamel (the lesion must still be visible when dry).

Code 3: Localized Enamel Breakdown due to Caries with no Visible Dentin or Underlying Shadow

The tooth viewed may have a clear carious opacity (white spot lesion) and/or brown carious discoloration which is wider than the natural fissure/ fossa that is not consistent with the clinical appearance of sound enamel. Once dried, there is carious loss of tooth structure at the entrance to, or within, the pit or fissure/fossa. This will be seen visually as evidence of demineralization [opaque (white), brown or dark brown walls] at the entrance to or within the fissure or pit, and although the pit or fissure may appear substantially and unnaturally wider than normal, the dentin is not visible in the walls or base of the cavity/discontinuity.

If in doubt, or to confirm the visual assessment, the WHO/CPI/PSR probe can be used gently across a tooth surface to confirm the presence of a cavity apparently confined to the enamel. This is achieved by sliding the ball end along the suspect pit or fissure and a limited discontinuity is detected if the ball drops into the surface of the enamel cavity/discontinuity.

Code 4: Underlying Dark Shadow from Dentin with or without Localized Enamel Breakdown

As a shadow of discolored dentin visible through an apparently intact enamel surface which may or may not show signs of localized breakdown (loss of continuity of the surface that is not showing the dentin). The shadow appearance is often seen more easily when the tooth is wet. The darkened area is an intrinsic shadow which may appear as grey, blue or brown in color. The shadow must clearly represent caries that started on the tooth surface being evaluated. If in the opinion of the examiner, the carious lesion started on an adjacent surface and there is no evidence of any caries on the surface being scored then the surface should be coded "0".

Code 3 and 4, histologically may vary in depth with one being deeper than the other and vice versa. This will depend on the population and properties of the enamel. For example more translucent and thinner enamel in primary teeth may allow the undermining discoloration of the dentin to be seen before localized breakdown of enamel. However, in most cases code 4 is likely to be deeper into dentin than code 3.

Code 5: Distinct Cavity with Visible Dentin

Cavitation in opaque or discolored enamel are exposing the dentin beneath. The tooth viewed wet may have darkening of the dentin visible through the enamel. Once dried, there is visual evidence of loss of tooth structure at the entrance to or within the pit or fissure—frank cavitation. There is visual evidence of demineralization at the entrance to or within the pit or fissure and in the examiner judgment dentin is exposed.

The WHO/CPI/PSR probe can be used to confirm the presence of a cavity apparently in dentin. This is achieved by sliding the ball end along the suspect pit or fissure and a dentin cavity is detected if the ball enters the opening of the cavity and in the opinion of the examiner the base is in dentin (in pits or fissures the thickness of the enamel is between 0.5 and 1.0 mm. The deep pulpal dentin should not be probed).

Code 6: Extensive Distinct Cavity with Visible Dentin

Obvious loss of tooth structure, the cavity is both deep and wide and dentin is clearly visible on the walls and at the base. An extensive cavity involves at least half of a tooth surface or possibly reaching the pulp.

Smooth Surface (Mesial And Distal)

This requires visual inspection from the occlusal, buccal and lingual directions.

Code 0: Sound Tooth Surface

There should be no evidence of caries (either no or questionable) change in enamel translucency after prolonged air drying. Surfaces with developmental defects, such as enamel hypoplasias; fluorosis; tooth wear (attrition, abrasion and erosion) and extrinsic or intrinsic stains will be recorded as sound.

Code 1: First Visual Change in Enamel

When seen wet there is no evidence of any change in color attributable to carious activity, but after prolonged air drying a carious opacity (white or brown lesion) is visible that is not consistent with the clinical appearance of sound enamel. This will be seen from the buccal or lingual surface.

Code 2: Distinct Visual Change in Enamel when Viewed Wet

There is a carious opacity or discoloration that is not consistent with the clinical appearance of sound enamel. This lesion may be seen directly when viewed from the buccal or lingual direction. In addition, when viewed from the occlusal direction, this opacity or discoloration may be seen as a shadow confined to enamel, seen through the marginal ridge.

Code 3: Initial Breakdown in Enamel due to Caries with no Visible Dentin

Once dried for approximately 5 seconds, there is distinct loss of enamel integrity, viewed from the buccal or lingual direction. If in doubt, or to confirm the visual assessment, the CPI probe can be used gently across the surface to confirm the loss of surface integrity.

Code 4: Underlying Dark Shadow from Dentin with or without Localized Enamel Breakdown

This lesion appears as a shadow of discolored dentin visible through an apparently intact marginal ridge, buccal or lingual walls of enamel. This appearance is often seen more easily when the tooth is wet. The darkened area is an intrinsic shadow which may appear as grey, blue or brown in color.

Code 5: Distinct Cavity with Visible Dentin

Cavitation in opaque or discolored enamel (white or brown) with exposed dentin in the examiner's judgment, if in doubt, or to confirm the visual assessment, the CPI probe can be used to confirm the presence of a cavity apparently in dentin. This is achieved by sliding the ball end along the surface and a dentin cavity is detected if the ball enters the opening of the cavity, and in the opinion of the examiner the base is in dentin.

Code 6: Extensive Distinct Cavity with Visible Dentin

Obvious loss of tooth structure, the extensive cavity may be deep or wide and dentin is clearly visible on both the walls and at the base. The marginal ridge may or may not be present. An extensive cavity involves at least half of a tooth surface or possibly reaching the pulp.

A simple decision tree is provided for applying the 7-code for classifying coronal tooth surfaces following the ICDAS criteria

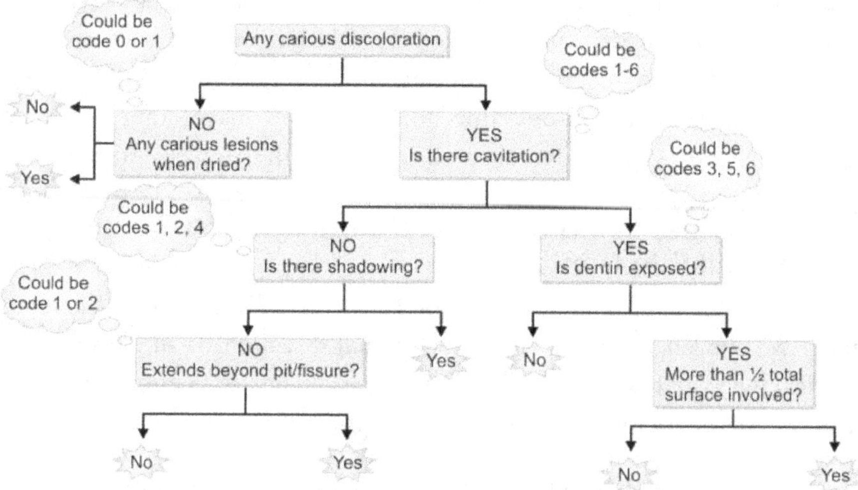

Figure 5: Flowchart

Caries-Associated with Restorations and Sealants (CARS) Detection Criteria

Since outer carious lesions adjacent to restorations are thought to be analogous with primary caries, the broad principles applied to the criteria for primary caries are also applied to CARS where relevant.

Code 0: Sound Tooth Surface with Restoration or Sealant

A sound tooth surface adjacent to a restoration/sealant margin, there should be no evidence of caries. Surfaces with marginal defects less than 0.5 mm in width, developmental defects, and extrinsic or intrinsic stains will be recorded as sound. Stained margins consistent with non carious and which do not exhibit signs consistent with demineralization should be scored as sound.

Code 1: First Visual Change in Enamel

When seen wet there is no evidence of any change in color attributable to carious activity, but after prolonged air drying an opacity or discoloration consistent with demineralization is visible that is not consistent with the clinical appearance of sound enamel.

Code 2: Distinct Visual Change in Enamel/Dentin Adjacent to a Restoration/Sealant Margin

If the restoration margin is placed on enamel, the tooth must be viewed wet. When wet, there is an opacity consistent with demineralization or discoloration that is not consistent with the clinical appearance of sound enamel and If the restoration margin is placed on dentin, discoloration that is not consistent with the clinical appearance of sound dentin or cementum is code 2.

Code 3: Carious Defects of < 0.5 mm with the Signs of code 2

Cavitation at the margin of the restoration/sealant less than 0.5 mm, in addition to either an opacity or discoloration consistent with demineralization that is not consistent with the clinical appearance of sound enamel or with a shadow of discolored dentin.

Code 4: Marginal Caries in Enamel/Dentin/Cementum Adjacent to Restoration/Sealant with Underlying Dark Shadow from Dentin

The tooth surface may have characteristics of code 2 and has a shadow of discolored dentin which is visible through an apparently intact enamel surface or with localized breakdown in enamel but no visible dentin. This appearance is often seen more easily when the tooth is wet and is a darkening and intrinsic shadow which may be grey, blue, orange or brown in color.

Code 5: Distinct Cavity Adjacent to Restoration/Sealant

Distinct cavity adjacent to restoration/sealant with visible dentin in the interfacial space with signs of caries as described in code 4, in addition to a gap > 0.5 mm in width or in those instances where margins are not visible, there is evidence of discontinuity at the margin of the restoration/ sealant and tooth substance of the dentin as detected by 0.5 mm ball-ended probe run along the restoration/sealant margin.

Code 6: Extensive Distinct Cavity with Visible Dentin

Obvious loss of tooth structure, the extensive cavity may be deep or wide and dentin is clearly visible on both the walls and at the base.

ICDAS Two-digit Coding Method

A two-number coding system is suggested to identify restorations/sealants with the first digit, followed by the appropriate caries code, e.g. a tooth restored with amalgam, which also exhibited an extensive distinct cavity with visible dentin would be coded 4 (for an amalgam restoration) and 6 (distinct cavity), an unrestored tooth with a distinct cavity would be 06. The suggested restoration/sealant coding system is as follows:[7]

- 0 = Sound, i.e. surface not restored or sealed (use with the codes for primary caries)

- 1 = Sealant, partial

- 2 = Sealant, full

- 3 = Tooth colored restoration

- 4 = Amalgam restoration

- 5 = Stainless steel crown

- 6 = Porcelain or gold or PFM crown or veneer

- 7 = Lost or broken restoration

- 8 = Temporary restoration

- 9 = Used for the following conditions

- 96 = Tooth surface cannot be examined; Surface excluded

- 97 = Tooth missing because of caries (tooth surfaces will be coded 97)

- 98 = Tooth missing for reasons other than caries (all tooth surfaces will be coded 98)

- 99 = Unerupted (tooth surfaces coded 99)

Root Caries

National Institutes of Health (NIH), consensus development conference on dental caries diagnosis and management concluded that there was insufficient evidence on the validity of clinical diagnostic systems for root caries.

Root caries are frequently observed near the cementoenamel junction (CEJ), although lesions can appear anywhere on the root surface. The color of the root lesions has been used as an indication of lesion activity. Active lesions have been described as being yellowish or light brown in color whereas arrested lesions appear darkly stained. However, color subsequently has been shown not to be a reliable indicator of caries activity. [15]

Codes for the Detection and Classification of Carious Lesions on the Root Surfaces

One score will be assigned per root surface. The facial, mesial, distal and lingual root surfaces of each tooth should be classified as follows:

Code E: If the root surface cannot be visualized directly as a result of gingival recession or by gentle air-drying, then it is excluded. Surfaces covered entirely by calculus can be excluded or the calculus can be removed prior to determining the surface.

Code 0: The root surface neither exhibits any unusual discoloration that distinguishes it from the surrounding or adjacent root areas nor does it exhibit a surface defect either at the CEJ or wholly on the root surface. The root surface may have a natural anatomical contour or the root surface may exhibit a definite loss of surface continuity or an anatomical contour not consistent with the caries process.

Code 1: There is a clearly demarcated area on the root surface or at the CEJ that is discolored but there is no cavitation present (loss of anatomical contour < 0.5 mm).

Code 2: There is a clearly demarcated area on the root surface or at the CEJ that is discolored (light/dark brown, black) and there is cavitation (loss of anatomical contour ≥; 0.5 mm) present.

New methods of caries detection are especially suitable for diagnosing early to moderate-stage lesions (ICDAS 1 to 4). Ability of each method to detect lesions on occlusal and proximal surfaces. Many of these new technologies work by measuring various optical characteristics of enamel that are affected by demineralization. Most use some form of light — from the blue green region to near-infrared region of the light spectrum.

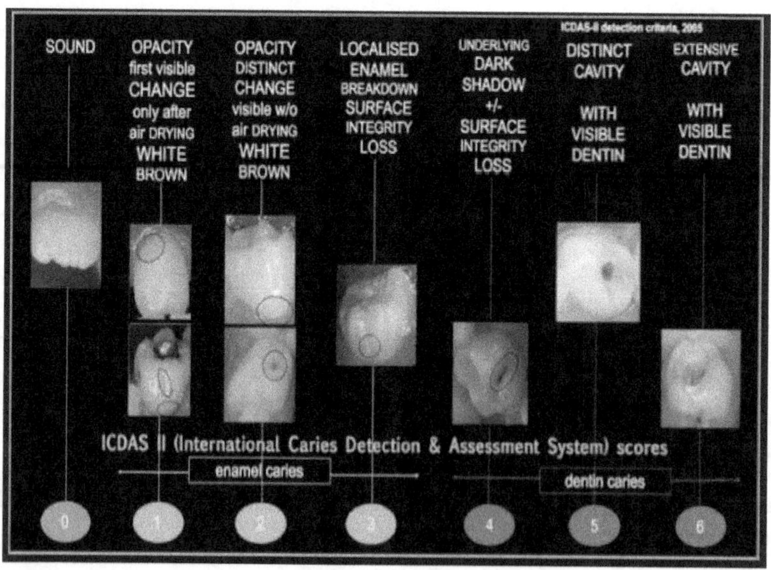

Figure 6: ICDAS II

Some measure reflectance (the amount of light reflected by the tooth surface in relation to the amount of incidental light), while others measure a combination of luminescence (the level of glow) and heat generated after a laser is shined on a tooth.

The methods based on **fluorescence** in the blue range are highly sensitive and can detect most initial lesions and combining this approach with a visual method might be a viable clinical alternative. Fluorescence in the infrared range has greater sensitivity for more severe lesions (ICDAS 2 to 4), but it is not as effective in diagnosing caries around restorations.

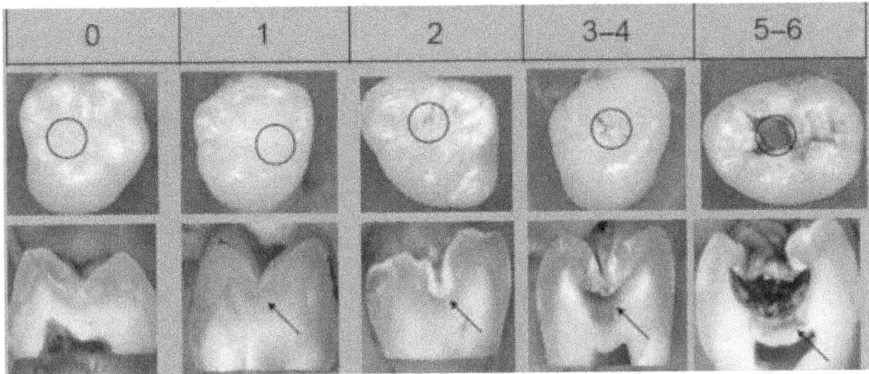

Figure 7: Clinical picture of ICDAS scale

While limited data show the tools that measure changes in reflectance from sound enamel to demineralized enamel can detect very early lesions (ICDAS 2 to 4), they may offer advantages that include minimal dilution of the light signal and insensitivity to the presence of bacteria.

Analyses of luminescence (glow) and thermal behaviour (heat) from the tooth are the basis of one technology. Some evidence indicates this system performs well in detecting enamel caries on occlusal surfaces and underneath sealants.

Methods that use transmission of light through the tooth structures perform similarly to bitewing radiographs in detecting approximal and occlusal caries when the lesions extend into dentin (ICDAS 3 and 4). These methods place a light on one surface and observe the area from a different surface.

ICDAS Lesion Severity		Activity Status	
		Active	Arrested
0	Sound		
1	First visual change in enamel	In plaque stagnation area. Enamel appears opaque or "chalky white" and rough. Gingival bleeding may be present on lesions close to the gingival margin	Not in plaque stagnation area. Enamel appears translucent or shiny, may be white or brown and smooth. No gingival bleeding in lesions close to the gingival margin
2	Distinct visual change in enamel		
3	Localized enamel breakdown		
4	Underlying dark shadow from dentin	May have the same characteristics of active ICDAS 1, 2 and 3 lesions	No progression based on longitudinal follow up with radiographs
5	Distinct cavity with visible dentin	Enamel surrounding the cavity appears opaque or chalky white and rough. Exposed dentin is light yellow, soft	Enamel surrounding the cavity appears translucent or shiny, may be white or brown and smooth. Exposed dentin is dark and hard
6	Extensive distinct cavity with visible dentin		

Table 14: Difference between active and Arrested caries

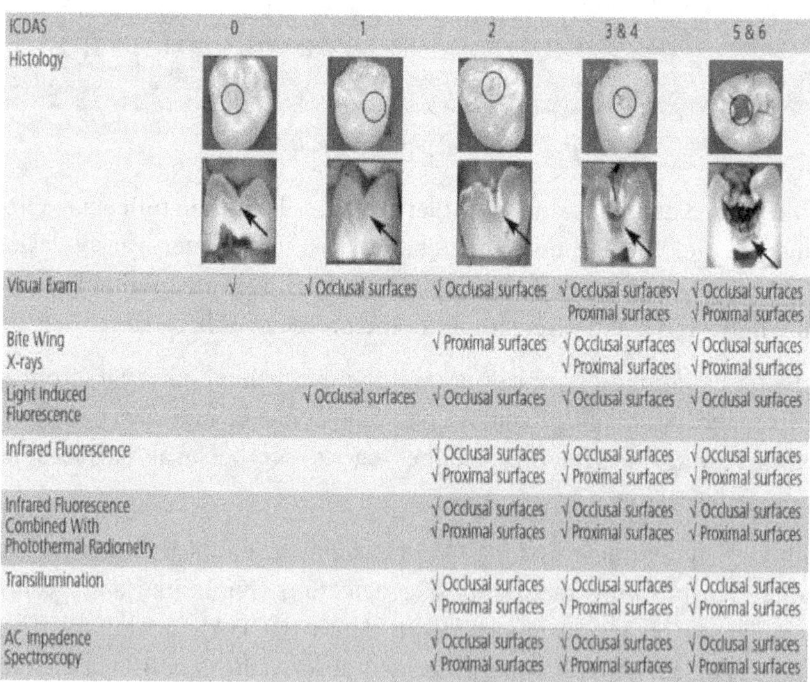

Figure 8: ICDAS Scoring

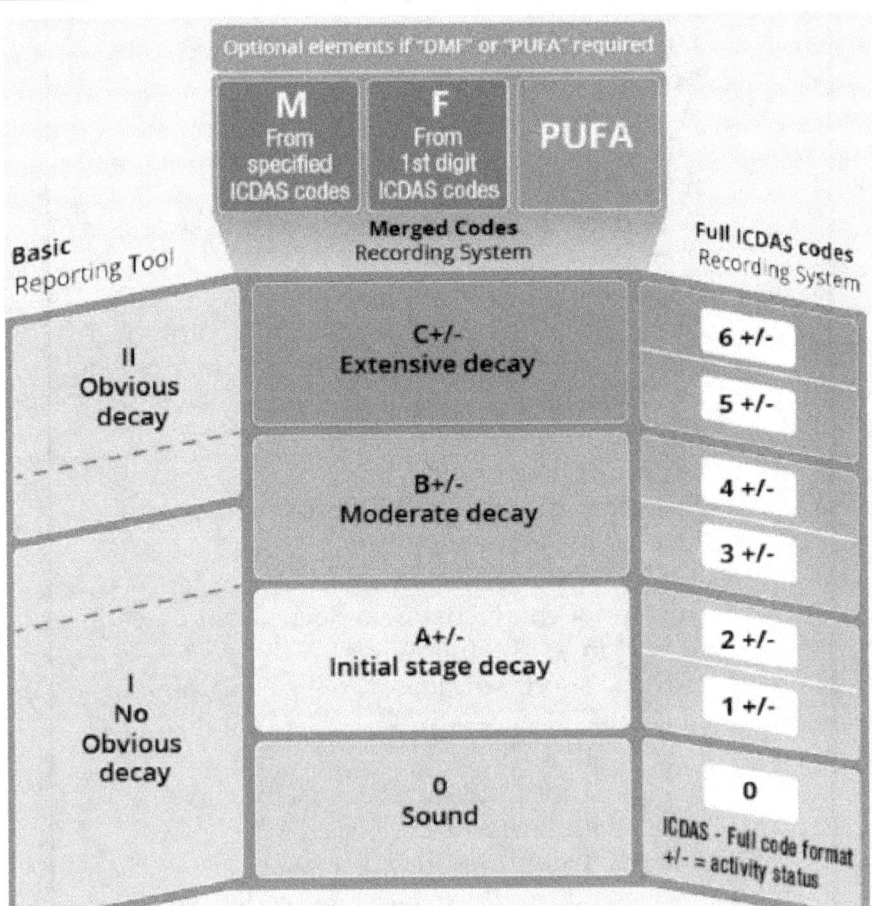

Figure 9: Scoring system

0	Un-restored or unsealed
1	Sealant, partial
	A sealant that does not cover all pits and fissures on a tooth surface
2	Sealant, full
	A sealant that covers all pits and fissure on a tooth surface
3	Tooth colored restoration
	In the opinion of the dentist, the tooth has a tooth colored (resin or glass–ionomer cement) restoration
4	Amalgam restoration
5	Stainless steel crown
6	Porcelain or gold or PFM crown or veneer
7	Lost or broken restoration
8	Temporary restoration
9	Tooth does not exist or other special cases. Used in as the following:
	9–6 = Tooth surface cannot be examined because of access problem to visualize the tooth surface
	9–7 = Tooth missing because of caries (all tooth surfaces are coded 97)
	9–8 = Tooth missing for reasons other than caries (all tooth surfaces are coded 98)
	9–9 = Un-erupted (all tooth surfaces care

Figure 10: Coding system

ICDAS in Literature

Pitts NB in 2013 provided an overview of the International Caries Detection and Assessment System (ICDAS) and its associated International Caries Classification and Management System (ICCMS(™)) to explain the evolution of these systems over the past decade and outline how they are being used for staging of the caries process in order to enable dentists to manage caries appropriately. It employs an evidence-based and preventively oriented approach, is a detection and assessment system classifying stages of the caries process on the basis of histological extent and activity, is designed for use in the four domains of clinical practice, education, research and public health and provides all stakeholders with a common language for staging caries. [16]

Over a decade ICDAS has evolved to comprise a number of approved, compatible 'formats', supports decision making at both individual and public health levels and has generated the ICCMS(™) to enable improved long-term caries outcomes. A range of further developments are in train, to assist with information capture and making clinical systems simpler and more practice friendly.

The study concluded that ICDAS helps in providing flexible and increasingly internationally adopted methods for classifying stages of the caries process and the activity status of lesions which can be incorporated into the ICCMS(™) . The ICCMS(™) provides option to dentists to integrate and synthesize tooth and patient information, including caries risk status, in order to plan, manage and review caries in clinical and public health practice.9

Till yester years, the epidemiological surveys have mainly focused on DMFT/DMFS to evaluate the prevalence of caries. But such studies rely on recording of cavitated lesions only. While ICDAS allows the recording of both cavitated and noncavitated lesions in continuum. various studies have evaluated the feasibility of using ICDAS II in epidemiological surveys by comparing it with the WHO criteria. In an in vivo study conducted by Braga MM et al (2009) in Brazil, 252 children were examined by two different examiners using ICDAS II or WHO criteria. Caries prevalence and examination time was calculated using both systems and it was observed that examination by ICDAS II took twice as long as by WHO criteria. It was concluded that ICDAS II, besides providing information on noncavitated caries lesions, can also generate data comparable to previous surveys which used the WHO criteria.

Studies have also shown good inter- and intraexaminer reproducibility and the accuracy of ICDAS II in detecting occlusal caries, especially in the outer half of the enamel. An in vitro study was done by Diniz MB et al (2009) using 163 molars that were assessed twice by two examiners using the ICDAS II scoring and were validated histologically using Ekstrand and Lussi histological scores. The inter- and intraexaminer kappa values were

0.51 and 0.58 respectively and it was concluded that ICDAS II presented good repro-ducibility and accuracy in detecting occlusal caries.

Momeni AJ et al (2010) evaluated intra- and interexaminer reproducibility of ICDAS II on occlusal caries diagnosis when different time intervals were allowed to elapse between examinations. Weighted kappa values for intra- and interexaminer reproducibility were 0.76 to 0.93 and it was observed that the time span did not have a major impact on assessing intra- and interexam-iner reproducibility. [17]

Shoaib L et al (2009) conducted an in vitro study to assess the validity and reproducibility of the ICDAS II criteria in primary teeth. The most advanced caries on the occlusal and approximal surfaces was recorded on 112 extracted primary molars followed by their sectioning and histological validation using the Downer and Ekstrand-Ricketts-Kidd (ERK) scoring systems and it was concluded that validity and reproducibility of the ICDAS II criteria were acceptable when applied to primary molar teeth.[18]

Surveys have been done to compare the ICDAS criteria with the other conventional methods of detecting, scoring and diagnosing dental caries.

Kuhnisch J et al (2008) compared the diagnostic outcome of the WHO criteria, ICDAS II criteria, laser fluorescence measurements and found good diagnostic potential of the ICDAS II criteria in comparison to the traditional WHO criteria such that ICDAS II proved helpful in detecting noncavitated caries lesions as well.[19] The study also emphasized the limited use of DIAGNOdent in field studies, when using ICDAS method for caries recording.

Another study by **Rodrigues JA et al (2008)** compared the performance of fluorescence-based methods, radio-graphic examination and ICDAS II on occlusal surfaces.[20] A total of 119 permanent molars were assessed using the laser fluorescence (LF and LFpen) and fluorescence camera (FC) devices, ICDAS II and bitewing radiographs (BW) followed by their histological validation. The sensitivities for dentine caries detection were 0.86 (FC), 0.78 (LFpen), 0.73 (ICDAS II), 0.51 (LF) and 0.34 (BW) and the specificities were 0.97 (BW), 0.89 (LF), 0.65 (ICDAS II), 0.63 (FC) and 0.56 (LFpen). Thus, it was concluded that LFpen, FC and ICDAS II presented better sensitivity and LF and BW better specificity. Also, ICDAS II combined with BW showed the best performance.

Diamanti I, Berdouses ED, Kavvadia K, Arapostathis KN, Reppa C, Sifakaki M, Panagopoulou in 2021*evaluated* the caries status of 5, 12 and 15-year-old Greek children, assess how disease parameters are related to socio-demographic indicators and identify relevant trends at the national level. 3702 children in total was randomly selected and examined clinically for caries (ICDAS II criteria). 7 Caries experience was outlined by adapting ICDAS0-6 criteria to the d/D component of the WHO dmf/DMF index configuration. Percentages (%) of caries experience-free children, of children with initial caries (ICDAS1-2), and the mean d1-2t/D1-2T, d3-6mft/D3-6MFT and d3-6mfs/D3-6MFS indices were calculated.

60.1%, 48.1%, and 34.7% of the 5, 12, and 15-year-old children, respectively, had no caries experience at the defect level (d3-6mft/D3-6MFT = 0). Initial lesions (ICDAS1-2) were detected in 17.7%, 19.3% and 17.4% of the 5, 12 and 15-year-olds, accordingly. Mean d1-2t/D1-2T was 0.93, 1.70, and 2.51, whereas mean d3-6mft/D3-6MFT was 1.48, 1.61, and 2.46 for the 5, 12, and 15-year-olds, respectively. Children with higher educated parents and 15-year-old urban residents exhibited significantly less caries experience at the defect level. Initial caries lesions presented a significantly higher probability of being detected in urban-residing 5- and 15-year-olds, while no consistent trend could be identified for parental education level. Caries prevalence and experience levels declined for all age groups in ten years.

The study concluded that Dental health of Greek children has improved disparities remain, calling for organised primary and secondary preventive interventions

Tassoker M. · Ozcan S. · Karabekiroglu S in 2020 compared the performance of visual inspection (ICDAS-II), laser fluorescence (DIAGNOdent pen), and the near-infrared transillumination technique (DIAGNOcam) in the detection of non-cavitated occlusal caries lesions under clinical and laboratory conditions in 90 third molar teeth planned for extraction. [21]

Ninety third molar teeth were firstly examined in clinical conditions, scored according to ICDAS-II criteria, and examined with DIAGNOdent pen and DIAGNOcam devices. After finishing the clinical examination, the teeth were re-evaluated shortly after the extractions with the same methods. Then, the teeth were sectioned for histological validation according to Downer's criteria. Sensitivity, specificity, accuracy, and area under the receiver operating characteristic (ROC) curves were calculated based on the histological results.

For the D0–D1–4 threshold, the area under the ROC curve values ranged between 0.754 and 0.881 for all systems. Sensitivity values ranged between 80.5 and 96.1%, and specificity values ranged between 61.5 and 84.6% for the three caries detection methods. Diagnocam had the best correlation value (0.616) according to histological observations and demonstrated a sensitivity rate of 96.1%, a specificity rate of 61.5%, and an accuracy rate of 91.1%. The study concluded that diagnocam was found to be the most effective method for the diagnosis of occlusal caries without cavitation in permanent molar teeth.

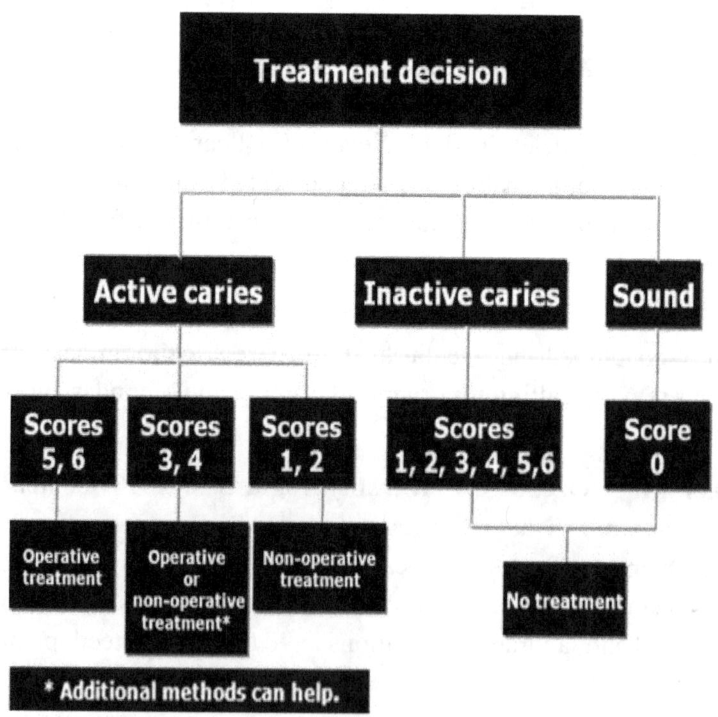

Figure 11: Flowchart depicting Treatment decision

Iceberg Of Dental Caries': Diagnostic Thresholds In Clinical Trials And Practic

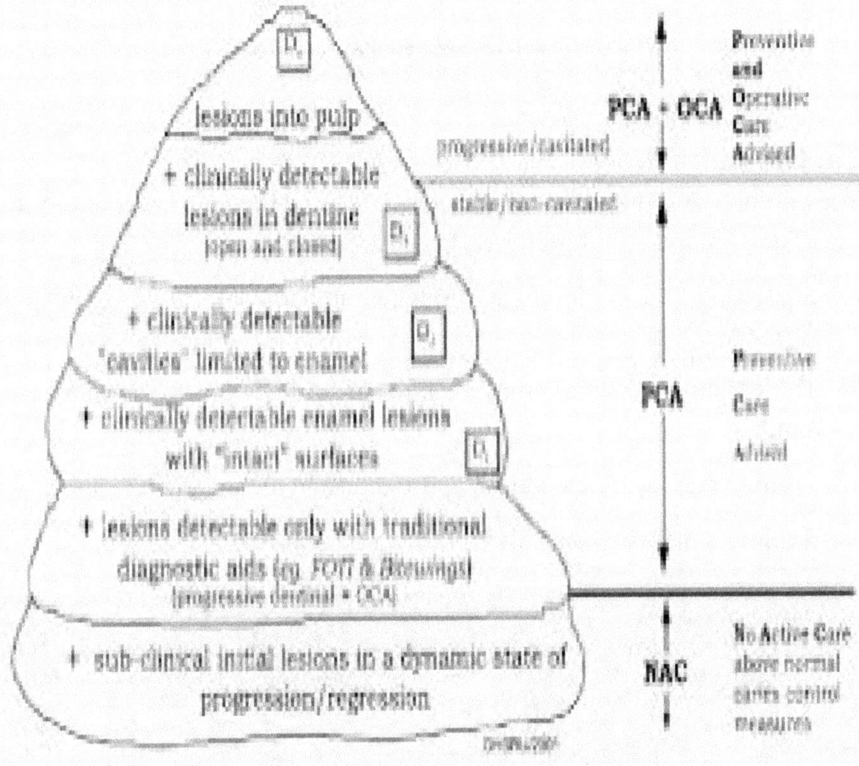

Figure 12: Iceberg Principle Of Dental Caries

The continuous process of caries has been represented by an iceberg as a metaphor to conceptualize dental caries. The iceberg represents the whole arrange of lesions and shows how traditional methods may leave undetected a large number of early lesions depending at which diagnostic threshold the methods are used

Visual Tactile Examination

Tactile Sensation

The explorer and the dental floss are used for tactile examination but the use of an explorer is not preferred because ;

1. Sharp tip of the explorer can produce traumatic defects on the enamel surface,

2. The cariogenic bacteria may be transferred from one tooth surface to another,

3. Probing may cause cavitation and fracture in the incipient lesions,

4. Explorers have low sensitivity resulting in undetected lesions.

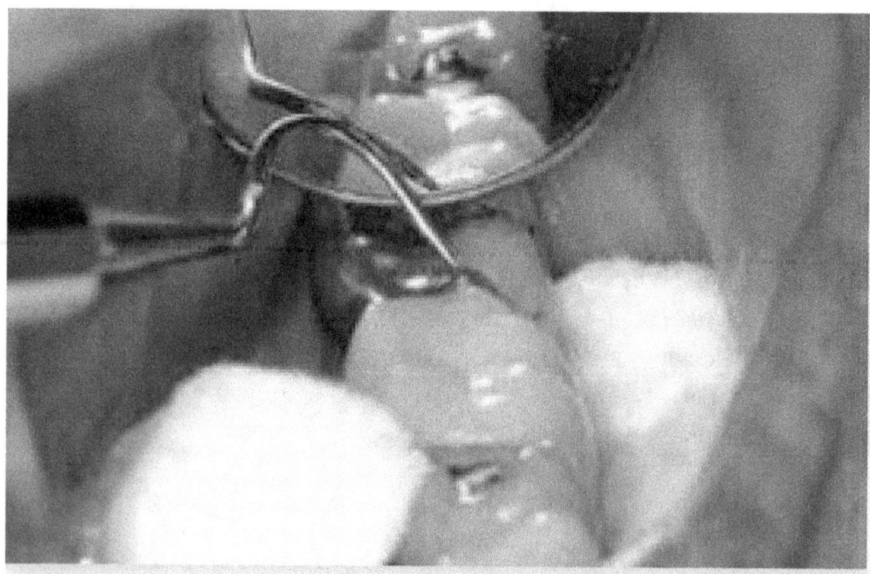

Figure 13: Tactile sensation

If the explorer catches or resists removal when moderate pressure is applied, and when this is accompanied by one of the following;

- Softness at the base of the lesion,

- Opacity adjacent to the pit or fissure,

- The enamel is softened adjacent to the pit and fissure, which can be concluded that the area is carious. Pickard, proposed the use of dental floss for the detection of caries when there is food packed between the teeth ,the floss is frayed when passed through the contact area, this might be the indication of caries .

Proximal caries has been very difficult to diagnose using the visual tactile method as 83% of cavitated proximal caries lesions were not detected using this method alone.

Gingival inflammation could thus be used as an additional diagnostic indicator for the presence or absence of cavitations in proximal surface.

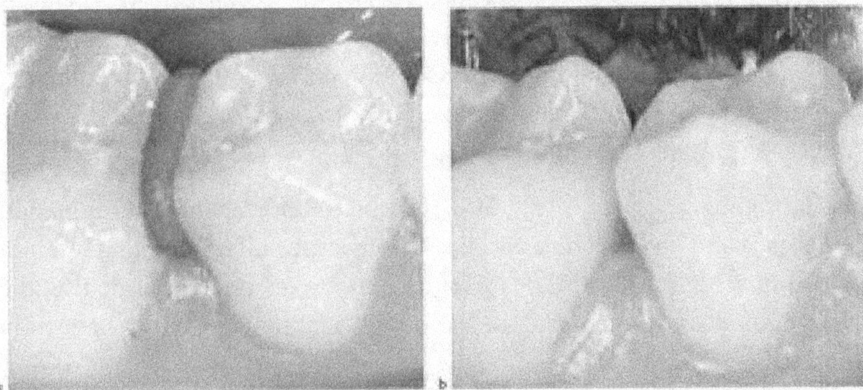

Figure 14: Tooth Separation With Elastics For Visualisation Of Caries

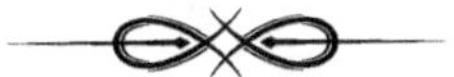

Radiography

Dental radiography is electromagnetic radiation, which has wavelengths between 0.01 to 10 nanometers which utilizes the fact that the absorption of the x-rays differs depending on what type of tissue they penetrate. The difference can be visualized by the use of different kind of detectors, analog, as well as digital. X-ray is especially useful for hard tissue diagnostics. Unlike the visual-tactile method, X-rays are potentially harmful, and should only be used when indicated.

Radiographs are useful for caries detection because caries causes demineralization of the tooth structure. Demineralized tooth structure attenuates the x-ray photons to a lesser extent than sound tooth structure. A minimum of 60% demineralization must occur before the lesion can be seen on a film-based radiograph.

Digital radiographs are in the 50-55% range. Radiographic examination has great value in detecting carious lesions especially when they are not clinically visible. In low caries population, as a result of fluoride use, the surface of enamel does not break down, making the caries detection harder.[22]

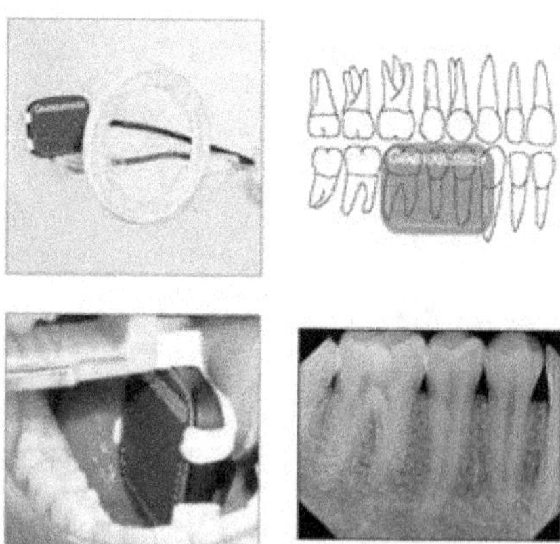

Figure 15: Intraoral Radiograph

Score	Criteria
0	No or slight change in enamel translucency after prolonged air-drying (5 seconds).
1	Opacity or discoloration hardly visible without drying, but visible after air-drying.
2	Opacity or discoloration visible even without air-drying.
3	Localized enamel breakdown in opaque or discolored enamel and/or grayish discoloration from the underlying dentin.
4	Cavitation in opaque or discolored enamel exposing the dentin.

Table 15: Criteria for ICDAS Scoring

Visual clinical examination according to Ekstrand et al 1997

Score	Criteria
0	No visible radiolucency.
1	Radiolucency in the enamel.
2	Radiolucency in the dentin, involving the surface or outer third of the dentin.
3	Radiolucency in the dentin, involving the middle third of the dentin.
4	Radiolucency in the dentin, involving the inner third of the dentin.

Table 16: Radiographic Examination According To Ekstrand et al. 1997

Bite Wing Projections:

Bitewing projections provide optimal visualization of proximal and occlusal caries in the posterior teeth. Periapical radiographs are appropriate for anterior proximal caries and its seen paralleling technique improves visibility of the lesion.

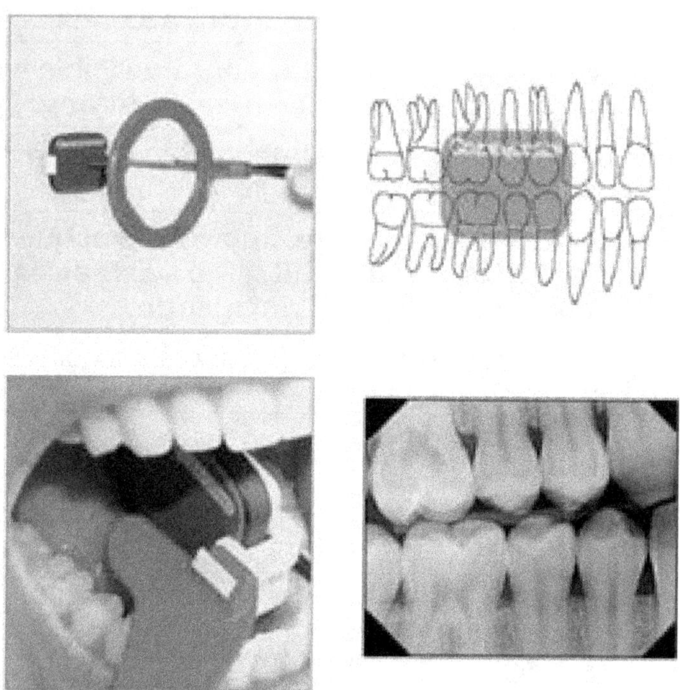

Figure 16: Bitewing Radiograph

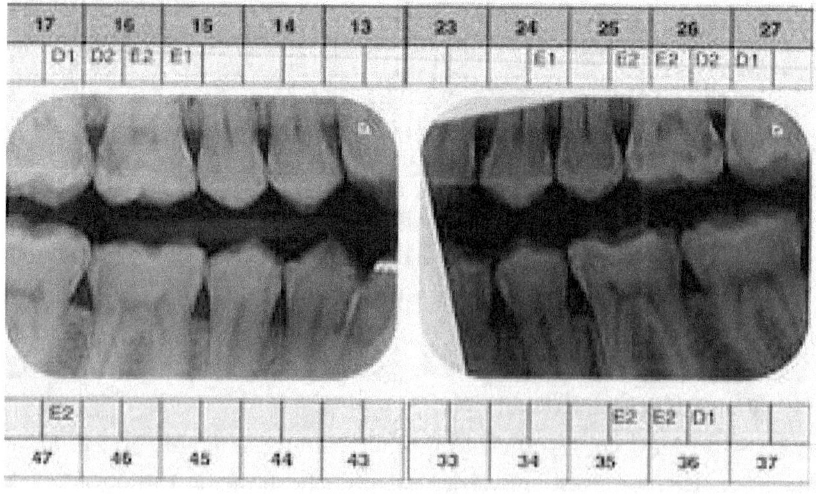

Figure 17: Bitewing Radiograph

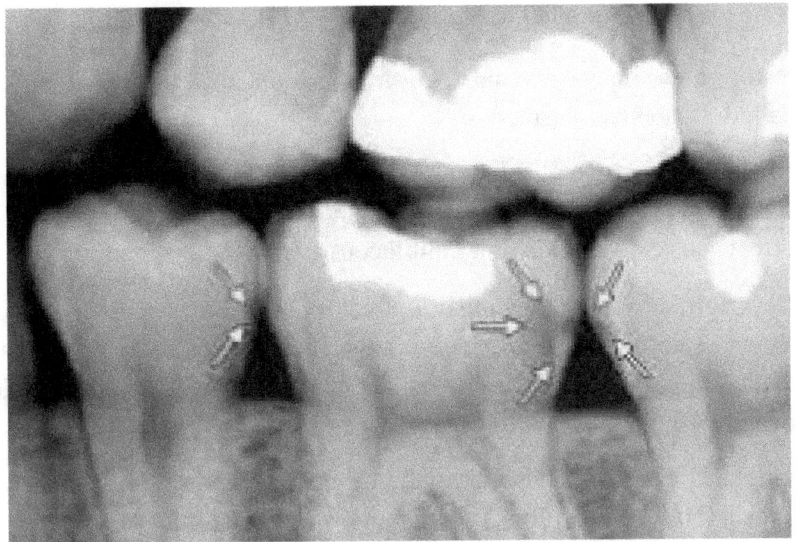

Figure 18: Bitewing Radiograph

Occlusal caries can often be detected on panoramic projections. Proximal dentin lesions are however more easily detected with X-ray compared to the visual-tactile method. Combining the visual-tactile method with bitewing radiographs seems to yield higher sensitivity and specificity, compared to either method alone.

According to studies, bitewing radiography has been proven to be an effective method in the detection of proximal caries and hidden caries. In recent years, the incidence of such lesions has increased dramatically .

Limitations:

- Proximal contacts are overlapped,

- The lesion depth may appear to be increased due to angulation and this may lead to false diagnosis,

- Occlusal lesions may not be detected because of the superposition of the buccal and lingual cusps,

- The real cause of the radiolucency can't be determined whether it is due to caries, resorption or wear,

- The superficial demineralization of the buccal and lingual surfaces may seem like proximal caries,

- Active and arrested caries can't be distinguished in the radiographs,

- Radiographs may give false positive results due to a phenomenon called "Mach band effect".

  In this perceptual phenomenon, the contrast between the dark and lighter areas has increased, resulting in a dark demarcation band. This effect causes formation of a radiolucent area in dentin enamel junction,

- Cervical burn out is another optical phenomenon where a wedge shaped radiolucent area is seen between the bone and the cemento-enamel junction. This effect is due to tissue density and the low penetration of X-rays at the cervical region.

Despite the disadvantages, radiographs are the most commonly used diagnosis tool and with the development of new techniques many of the problems are solved .

Scores for radiographical classification of lesion severity

Score	Criteria
0	no radiolucency
1	radiolucency in outer ½ of the enamel
2	radiolucency in inner ½ of the enamel ± EDJ
3	radiolucency limited to the outer 1/3 of dentine
4	radiolucency reaching the middle 1/3 of dentine
5	radiolucency reaching the inner 1/3 of dentine, clinically cavitated
6	radiolucency into the pulp, clinically cavitated

Figure 19: Scoring For Radiographical Classification

Digital Imaging Radiography

It s a form of radiography that uses X-ray - sensitive plates to capture data and then immediately transferring it to a computer system without the use of an intermediate cassette.

Advantages:

Immediate image preview;

Elimination of film processing steps;

Less radiation;

Wider dynamic range, which reduces the chances of over- and under-exposure;

Ability to apply special image processing techniques that enhance overall display quality of the image.

No significant difference between digital and conventional radiographic modalities in the detection of non-cavitated interproximal caries was observed by **Abesi *et al*** and **Abreu *et al.*,** and Syriopoulos et al who concluded that the diagnostic accuracy of digital systems is comparable with that of dental films, and the main contributing factor for correct diagnosis depends on the ability of dentists, but not the imaging modality.[23]

El-Samarrai and Misbah compared the diagnosis of an initial carious lesion by clinical and conventional radiographic methods in comparison to direct digital radiography. They concluded for both dentitions, the direct digital radiographs were more precise in the detection of decayed surfaces compared to both clinical and conventional radiographic examinations. [24]

Pontual *et al.* showed that the performance of the three intraoral storage phosphor plate digital systems was similar to that of the conventional film for detection of approximal enamel caries, and the histological depth of enamel caries was not significantly correlated with radiographic measurements.[25]

One important advance with digital radiology was the introduction of caries detection software, **Logicon Caries Detector™** Software (Kodak Dental Systems, Atlanta, GA), for assisting in the diagnosis of interproximal caries.[26] It has the ability to locate and classify proximal caries, indicating the depth of caries penetration.

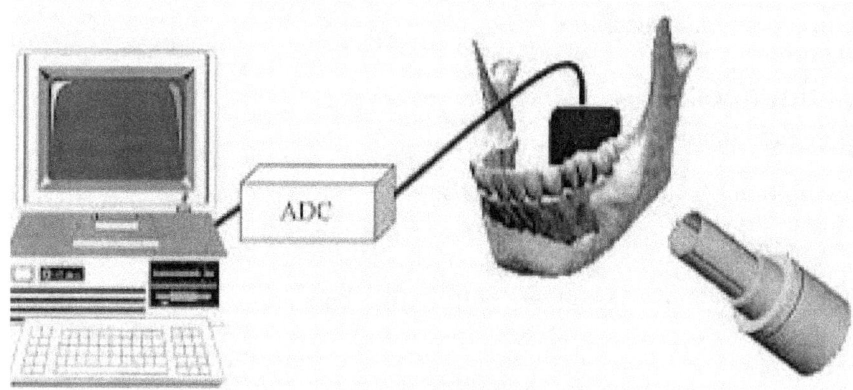

Figure 20 : Digital Radiography

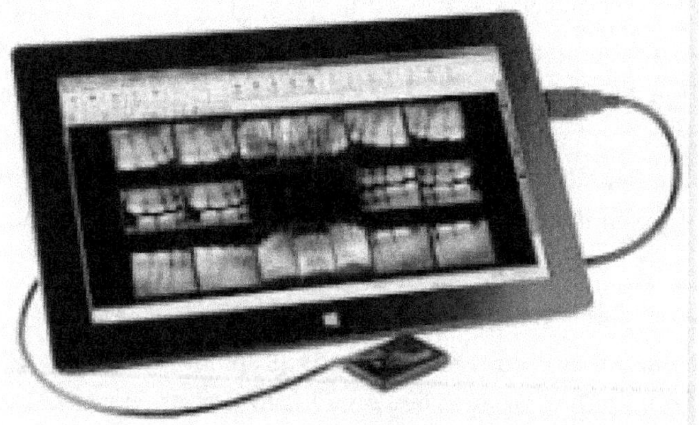

Figure 21: Digital Radiography

It has been offered as potential to increase the diagnostic yield of dental radiographs. It has manifested itself in subtraction radiography. A digital radiograph is comprised of a number of pixels where each pixel carries a value between 0 and 255, with 0 being black and 255 being white. The values in between represent shades of grey which can be quickly appreciated that a digital radiograph, with a potential of 256 grey levels has significantly lower resolution than a conventional radiograph that contain millions of grey levels.

Sensitivities and specificities of digital radiographs being significantly lower than those of regular radiographs when assessing small proximal lesions. However, digital radiographs offer the potential of image enhancement by applying a range of algorithms, some of which enhance the white end of the grey scale (such as Rayleigh and hyperbolic logarithmic probability) and others the black end (hyperbolic cube root function).

Digital radiographs offer a decrease in radiographic dose and thus offer additional benefits than diagnostic yield. Digital images can also be archived and replicated with ease.

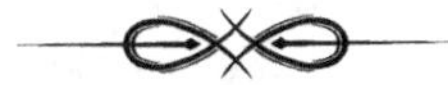

Xeroradiography

This technique uses the xeroradiographic copying process for recording images produced by X-rays. Xeroradiography is twice as sensitive as D-Speed films. This technique offers the opportunity of edge enhancement. Edge enhancement helps distinguishing the areas of different densities at the margins or edges For many years, xeroradiography was considered as a promising technique for caries detection but according to recent studies, it is regarded equivalent to E-Speed films used in conventional radiography.

It is a highly accurate electrostatic imaging technique that uses a modified xerographic copying process to record images produced by diagnostic X-rays. The process was invented and first used in 1937.

The most common application of xeroradiography in medical field is mammography, but it has also been successfully applied to imaging other body parts such as the skull, larynx, respiratory tract, TMJ, mandible, paraosseous soft tissues, and dental structures.

In 1955, the first recorded use of xeroradiography for alveolar structures took place. It was a lateral oblique view of the mandible.

Advantage :

Simultaneous evaluation of multiple tissues i.e. tissues with different thickness and densities can be easily viewed under one film.

It has excellent characteristics of the forces around the electrostatic charges, which form the latent image i.e. it provides a high-resolution images.

No special skills are required for office copying machine, even more so is the   xeroradiographic process.

Furthermore, dark room requirements are unnecessary, and the entire xeroradiographic process may be completed within 60 sec. The process also allows multiple copies simultaneously. It is the most cost effective method compared to either automatic processing or manual processing.

Periapical xeroradiographs were made using a smaller plate when compared with the plate size of conventional X-ray film.

It shows a well-defined and a sharp delineated bone details as well as soft tissue imaging on the same picture. These features offer advantage orthognathic surgery and in cephalometrics tracing especially in children.[27]

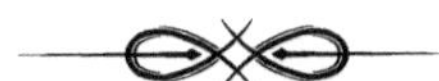

Modified Projection Techniques In Infants, Mentally Disabled Children , Children With Gag Reflex And Handicapped Children

Modified Projection Techniques:

Radiographs being a valuable tool are essential to diagnose oral diseases and to timely monitor the development of dentofacial structures and the results of the treatment outcomes. Because each patient is unique, initially a proper medical and dental history of the patient is required to determine the need for dental radiograph along with a complete clinical examination, and assessing the patient's vulnerability to environmental factors that affect oral health.

There are certain modifications for taking radiographs in infants, in young and handicapped children, children with gag reflex, and in special cases.

Intraoral radiographs may be made with the parent or guardian holding the films in place and use of film holding devices such as bite blocks or a hemostat extended through a rubber stopper may also be employed to retain the film.

In addition a film can be retained with the patient's occlusion, thus not being dependent on digital fixation.

In Infants:

An infant below 3 years of age, it is always recommended to use size 0 intraoral periapical films for the exposures to diagnose dental caries.

With the help of digital pressure, it becomes very difficult for the child to hold the film especially for maxillary molars. Similarly, the mandibular molar films and the bitewing radiographs impinge on the sublingual tissues thus causing irritation of the tissues.

Young children usually experience difficulty while taking a radiograph. In such cases, it becomes necessary to take parental help in which the parent is asked to hold the film or to hold both the child as well as the film. Both of them are asked to face in the same direction, and the patients head is stabilized with the parents shoulder and the radiograph is taken.

Mentally Disabled Children:

For patients with limited ability, to control film position, an intraoral film with bitewing tabs is used for all bitewing and periapical radiographs. An 18-inch length of floss is attached through a hole made in the tab (to facilitate retrieval of the film).

The patient should wear a lead apron with a thyroid shield, and anyone who helps hold the patients and films or sensor should wear lead - lined apron and gloves.

Children With Gag Reflex

Child may express his apprehension by an increased tendency to gag. It is necessary to acquaint the patient thoroughly with the radiographic procedure prior to filming. One of the most effective methods of reducing gagging is a distraction.

The child is asked to concentrate intensely on something spatially removed from the oral cavity. The task may be to raise one leg, and his toes, make a fist or hold his breath. The best time to perform the examination in the morning when the individual is well rested, rather than in the afternoon or evening.Also, it has been observed that the chance of gagging is reduced when the stomach is empty or half filled.

Pharmacological techniques for managing gag response include the use of sedative and topical anesthetic, phenothiazine derivatives, antihistamines, barbiturates, and nitrous oxide. For temporary relieving the gag reflex, use of local anesthetics such as xylocaine or dyclone in topical or rinse form is helpful.

General anesthesia is generally not considered as an approach for obtaining radiographs. Film size positioning and manner of placement may also be varied to accommodate the child who gags during radiography. Children have smaller jaws, shallow lingual vestibule require the use of smaller films. It is sometimes useful to place posterior film toward the front of the mouth initially and allow the child to move the film posteriorly into position himself.

Handicapped Children:

Many mentally handicapped children will not allow an intraoral film to be placed in their mouths. Intraoral radiographs of these children are usually obtained with the parent holding the film in position. A holding device that fixes the film in position while the patient occludes is more effective than trying to hold the film by digital placement.

Such patients cannot or will not open their mouth for radiographic procedures. In these cases, extraoral radiographs like panoramic, lateral jaw or 45° projections are used. Holding intraoral holder at times becomes difficult in handicapped children or young patients, wherein Rinn Snap-A-Ray is used instead of the use of conventional holders.

With the help of these modifications holding the film in the oral cavity becomes easier in handicapped and young children.

Modification in Film Packets and Holder Film packets can be modified in patients to reduce the anxiety level or to minimize the local discomfort and gagging associated with the placement of the film. This modification includes the bending of the film (occlusal), using the smallest possible film or either bending of the corners of the film to decrease the irritation especially in the sublingual area of the oral cavity.

Lewis *et al.* suggested the use of cotton rolls, which are taped with the packet of the film for maintaining the plane of the film.

For patients with gagging reflex, handicapped children or young children certain modifications of the film or film holder position are advocated. One technique includes the "reverse" bitewing in which the film is placed in the buccal vestibule, and the beam is directed through the jaws from the opposite side of patient's head.

Alternative To Intraoral Periapical Radiographs:

Extraoral techniques may be a good and reliable alternative when it is not possible or practical due to many factors, e.g. handicapped children, young patients or patient with a gag reflex.

The most common and frequently used substitute for intraoral radiography includes lateral jaw or lateral oblique and the panoramic films.

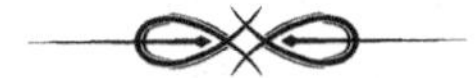

Novel Methods For Caries Detection

Digital detectors

- Charged couple device (CCD)
- Complementary metal oxide semiconductor
- Photo Stimulable Phosphor plate (PSP).

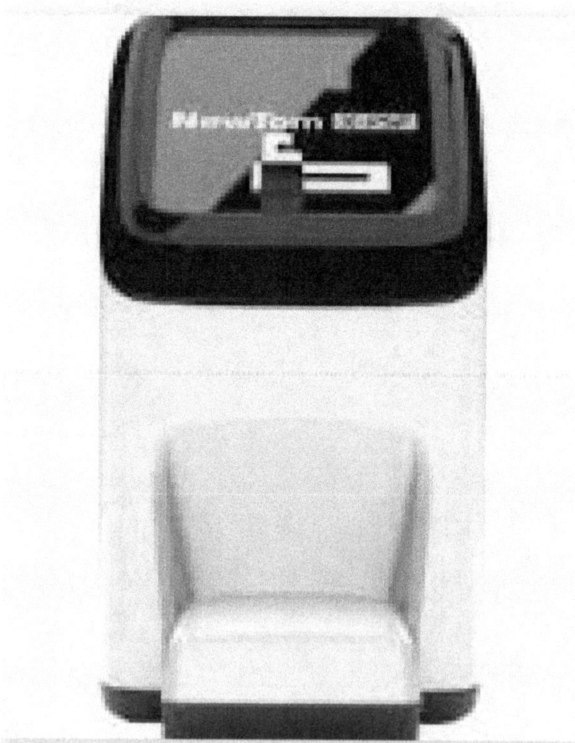

Figure 22: Digital Detectors

Digital Image Enhancement

Resolution of unenhanced digital image is lower than radiographs

- Range of gray shades is limited to 256, whereas in a radiographic film, over 1 million shades of gray appear

- Contrast can be digitally enhanced using a mathematical rule often decided by the algorithm/filter

- They are not practically used because they are very time-consuming.

Subtraction Radiography

This technique is extensively used for detection of caries and assessment of bone loss in periodontology . Digitalization is done by taking a picture of the radiograph with a high-quality video camera. This image is transferred to a computer imaging device named as digitizer. Two standardized radiographs exposed to same amounts of beam are superimposed using a software. The difference between the two images looks as dark bright areas .

Digital Imaging

Digital image is an image composed of a series of sensors and pixels distributed orderly. The advantages of digital imaging over conventional radiography is as follows:

The radiation dose is approximately 60-90% lower. The image receptor is often larger, image is immediately available, image can be electronically transferred, magnification, contrast, brightness can be adjusted. There is no need for processing solutions, protecting the environment and lowering the costs.

In order to be seen in the radiographs, there must be 40% of demineralization in the lesions. This means that detection of deeper lesions is significantly harder compared with superficial lesions . In an in vitro study comparing the capacity of conventional radiographic imaging with digital imaging systems in detection of proximal caries, it was concluded that these two systems provided similar results, showing no significant difference over another. It is highly recommended to use digital imaging as the radiation dose is significantly lower.

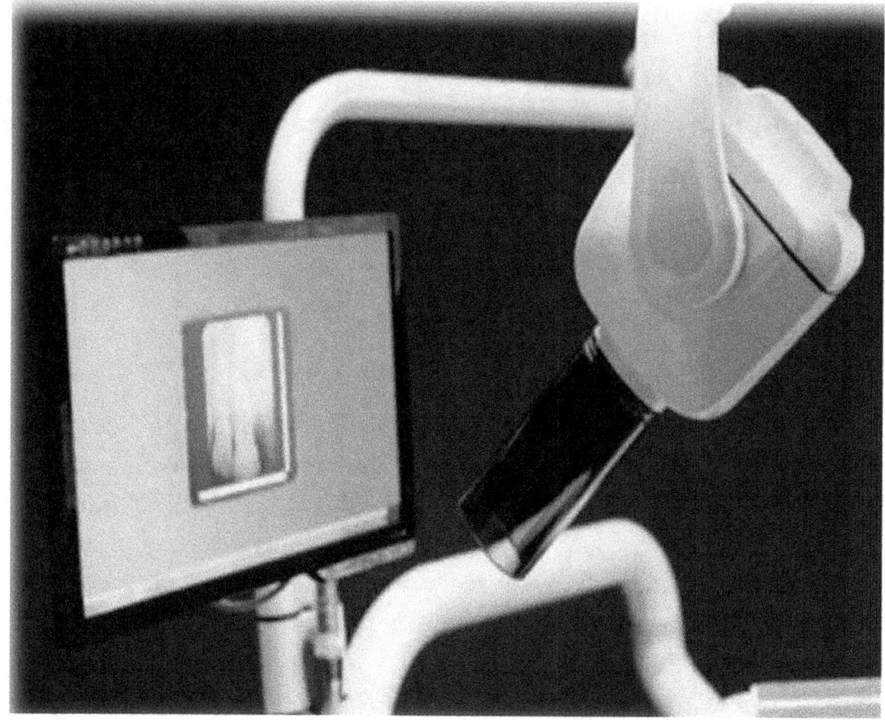

Figure 23: Digital Imaging

Subtraction Radiography

It is a technique by which structured noise is reduced to increase the detectability of changes in the radiographic pattern. Subtraction images can be obtained from photographic, electronic, and digital methods. Other methods have disadvantages such as inability to produce correct projection geometry and improper density and contrast.

Valizadeh *et al* showed that digital subtraction images have the potential to measure the depth of proximal caries; however, no significant difference was observed with histopathologic evaluation. [28]

Park *et al.* also demonstrated that digital subtraction radiography from single radiographic image of artificial caries was highly efficient in the detection of dental caries compared to the data from simple digital radiograph. [29]

Paymani *et al.* showed that DSR can be used as a specialized and precise method in the diagnosis of Class III caries.[30]

Digital Subtraction Radiography:

It distinguishes small differences between subsequent radiographs that otherwise would have remained unobserved because of over projection of anatomical structures or differences in density that are too small to be recognized by the human eye.

A digital bitewing radiograph is taken and later a second radiograph of exactly the same region is produced with identical exposure time, tube current, and voltage. By subtracting gray values for each coordinate of the first radiograph from equivalent coordinate of second, a subtraction image is obtained .

If no changes have occurred, the result of subtraction is zero. Nonzero result will be obtained in case of onset or progression of demineralization. It is not yet routinely applied in clinical caries detection due to difficulty of image registration

USES :

Assessment of the progression,

Arrest, or regression of caries lesions

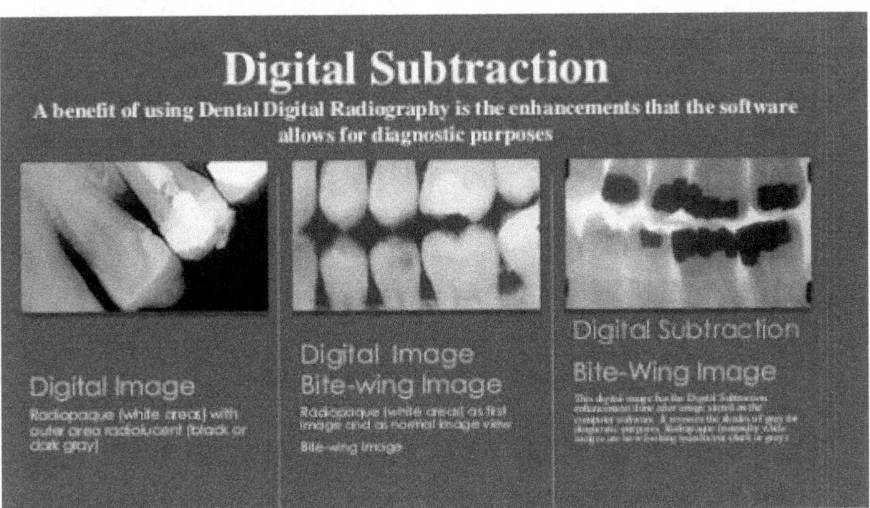

Figure 24 : Digital Subtraction

Principle: The basic premise of subtraction radiology is that two radiographs of the same object can be compared using their pixel values where pixels of first object is subtracted from the second image. If there is no change, the resultant pixel will be scored 0; any value that is not 0 must be attributable to either the onset or progression of demineralisation, or regression. When there is caries regression, the outcome will be a value above zero (increase in pixel values). In case of caries regression, the result is opposite and the outcome will be a value below zero (decrease in pixel values).

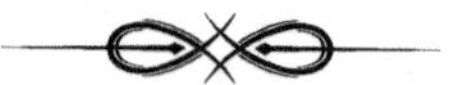

Specialized Radiographic Techniques

Computed Tomography (CT)

It was invented by Hounsfield in 1973 and is considered as a technical break-through, well-known medical technique for the non-destructive examination of internal structures and its introduction to dentistry has been innovative as it provides true three-dimensional (3D) imaging. It is also known as CAT scanning (computed axial tomography). The attenuation of an X-ray beam in the body is used in conventional radiography to project a shadow onto an image receptor where shadowgraphs record a two-dimensional (2D) representation of a three-dimensional (3D) object.[31]

Small lesions are therefore not readily identified because of overlapping and underlying anatomy, image distortion occurs because of unequal magnification effects and low contrast masses are poorly delineated since scatter contributes substantially to the image data. It is a radiographic technique that blends the concept of thin layer radiography (tomography) with computer synthesis. CT is a digital and mathematical imaging technique that creates tomographic sections where the tomographic layer is not contaminated by blurred structures from adjacent anatomy. It enables differentiation and is a non-invasive procedure.

CT examinations are quicker and more patient friendly. It is mainly indicated for investigations of intracranial diseases, preoperative assessment of maxillary alveolar bone height and thickness before inserting implants, investigations of suspected intracranial and spinal cord damage investigation and assessment of fractures involving the orbits and nasoethmoidal complex, cranial base and cervical spine fractures, tumor staging-assessment of site, size and extent of benign and malignant tumors' investigations of tumors and tumor-like discrete swelling intrinsic and extrinsic to the salivary glands and for the investigation of the temporomandibular joint (TMJ).

It eliminates superimposition of images of structures outside the area of interest; normal hidden surfaces can be examined in detail. It has the ability to rotate images and to add or subtract structural components permits relationships to be studied. Structural relationships of hard and soft tissues can be observed directly.

In CT imaging the effect of blurring is much greater than in conventional radiographic systems. The detail of a computed tomographic image is not as fine as that obtainable on other radiographs. Furthermore, the metallic objects such as fillings produce marked streak artifacts across the CT image. The equipment is very expensive.

Clinical application of CT in children includes diagnosis of neonatal maxilla and disorders involving the auditory ossicles and TMJ, provides a detailed view of the dental arches and positioning of the supernumerary teeth and gives idea about the extent of the cyst and tumors can be identified. In orthodontic cases, both skeletal as well as a dental relationship can be assessed. Proper evaluation of the trauma involving the face can be made with the use CT

Cone-beam CT (CBCT) is a new application of CT that generates 3D data at lower cost.

Van Daatselaar *et al.* carried out an *in vitro* observer study of the detection of interproximal caries by local CT, and it was observed that vertically reformatted CT slices obtained with local CT performed significantly better radiographs in visually detecting caries than conventional two-dimensional digital.[32] An in vitro observer study of the detection of interproximal caries by local CT was conducted for Detection of caries by means of conventional two-dimensional (2D) digital radiography and by two CT modalities was compared. Ground truth was obtained from histological examination of the sectioned teeth. Twenty-three extracted teeth (46 surfaces) were placed in groups of six in two dry mandibles. The observers (n=10) scored the proximal surfaces for the presence of caries on a 1-5 confidence scale. Data analysis used analysis of variance (a General Linear Model). Observer and method were entered into the model as within-subject variables and lesion depth was entered as a between-subjects variable.

The analysis showed observer, method and lesion depth effects as well as several interaction effects to be significant. Observers performed significantly better with the vertically reformatted CT slices than with conventional radiographs (P=0.025). Furthermore, there were significant differences between observers, and several interactions were found to be significant. This means that although the reformatted slices performed best overall, this performance differed significantly depending on observer and on lesion depth.

The study concluded that Vertically reformatted CT slices obtained with local CT performed significantly better than conventional 2D digital radiographs in visually detecting caries. Axial slices did not perform better than conventional radiographs. When vertically reformatted slices are used, local CT is a promising tool for the detection of interproximal caries.

Young *et al.* observed that dentists were able to detect dentinal proximal-surface caries using 3DX high-resolution CBCT images compared with CCD images when compared to occlusal dentinal caries.

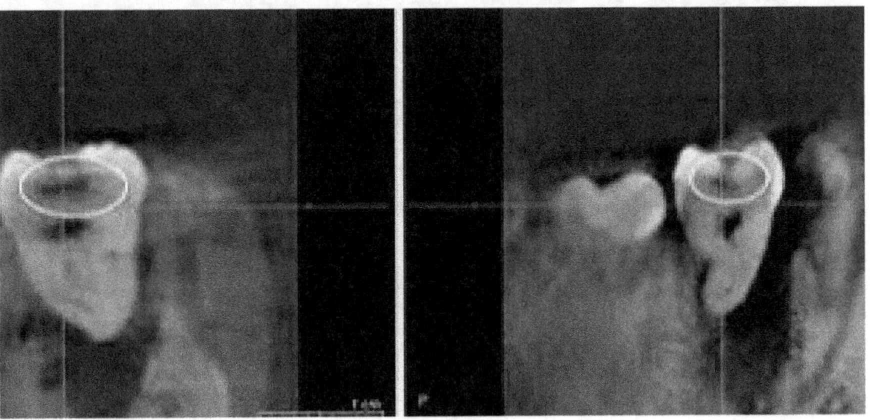

Figure 25: CT

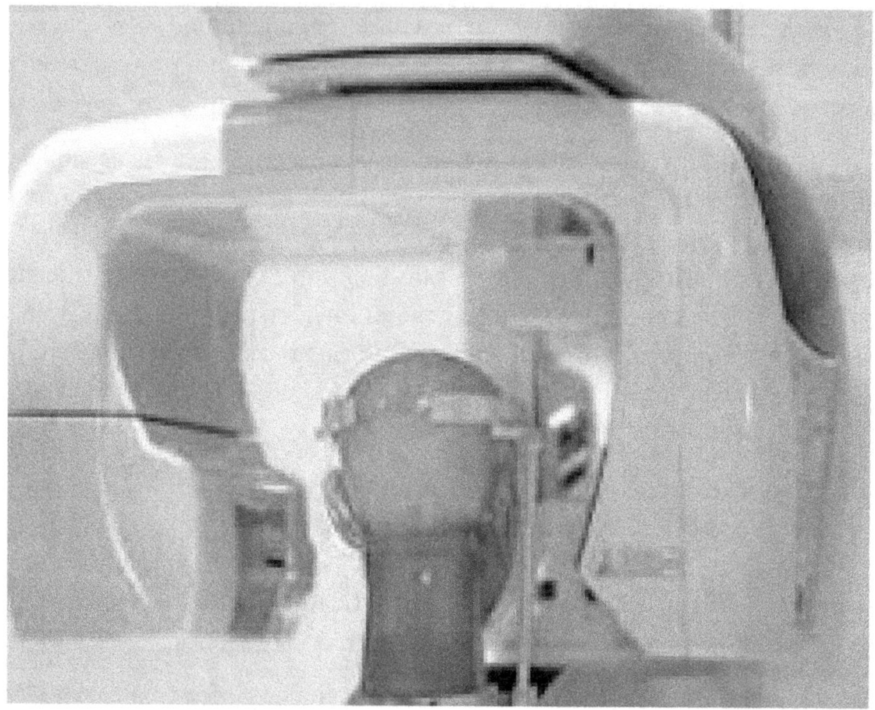

Figure 26A: CBCT IN CARIES

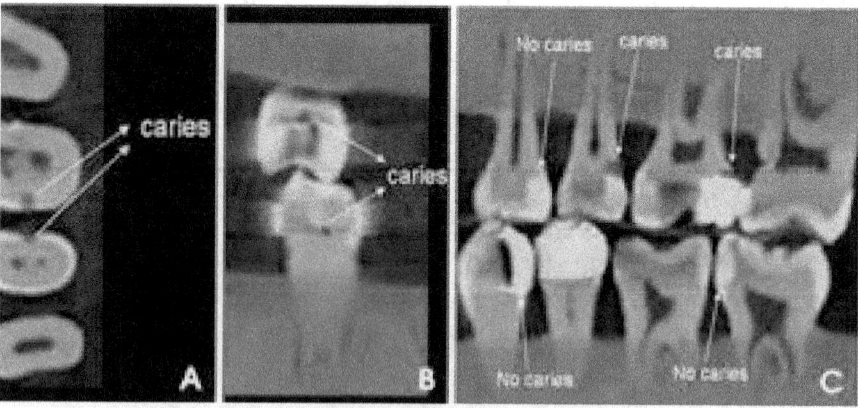

Figure 26 B: CBCT IN CARIES

CBCT In Children

Cone-beam CT (CBCT) is a new application of CT that generates 3D data at lower cost. It is also called as dental volumetric tomography, cone-beam volumetric tomography, dental CT, and cone beam imaging is a recent technology initially developed for angiography in 1982 and subsequently applied to maxillofacial imaging. It is only since the late 1980s that it has become possible to produce clinical systems that are both inexpensive and small enough to be used in the dental office.

The principal feature of CBCT is that multiple planar projections are acquired by rational scan to produce a volumetric dataset from which inter-relational images can be generated.

Cone-beam scanners use a 2D digital array providing an area detector rather than a linear detector as CT does. This is combined with a 3D X-ray beam with circular collimation so that the resultant beam is in the shape of a cone, hence the name "cone beam." Because the exposure incorporates the entire region of interest (ROI), only one rotational scan of the gantry is necessary to acquire enough data for image reconstruction.

As CBCT requires only a single scan for capturing the necessary data the time required for CBCT scanning is substantially less (<30 sec) as compared to conventional CT. CBCT data reconstruction and viewing is performed on a personal computer. Also, some manufacturers provide software with extended functionality mainly requires for orthodontic analysis and for implant placement.

CBCT can be used in pediatric patients having malocclusions and craniofacial anomalies, including cleft lip and palate. It is also proven to be helpful for the proper assessment and correct determination of the position of the unerupted teeth especially for the canines in upper arch and to determine the extent of root resorption. CBCT also provide a proper relationship between the dentition and for assessment of treatment planning and its outcome.This technology has limitations related to the cone beam projection geometry, detector sensitivity, and contrast resolution that produce images that lack the clarity and utility of conventional CT images.

Firstly used in the early 90s to generate 3-dimensional projections of X-ray images, cone beam computed tomography (CBCT) has resulted in a large application in dentomaxillofacial imaging, even in children. CBCT uses ionizing radiation that may cause damage to the DNA, and children are at the greatest carcinogenesis risk due to their higher tissue radiosensitivity and their longer life expectancy compared to adults. [33]

Radiography is still the most recommended adjunct method in the diagnosis of clinically inaccessible approximal surfaces. The major drawback of bitewing radiography for caries diagnosis is that the clinical state of the surface cannot be determined; i.e. if cavitation has developed or the demineralized surface is still intact. Based on studies of the relationship between radiographic lesion depth and clinical cavitation in approximal surfaces, a threshold for operative treatment decision has been suggested when a lesion is observed radiographically more than one-third into dentine.

However, the results from previous studies are contradictory and the majority of studies are ~25 years old. In addition, there are few longitudinal observational studies on the behaviour of dentinal carious lesions, particularly in adults.

It is an advanced 3-dimensional radiographic modality, which seems much more accurate than intra-oral modalities for displaying cavitation in approximal surfaces. Nonetheless, there are several drawbacks with CBCT, such as radiation dose, costs and imaging artefacts.

Bitewing radiography is, thus, still state-of-the-art as an adjunct in diagnosing carious lesions in clinically inaccessible approximal surfaces. The risk for cavitation is related to lesion depth, but new studies are needed in both child and adult populations to validate current thresholds for the operative treatment decision based on the radiographic lesion depth.

This technique is a new application of CT. The absorbed doses and the costs are significantly lower than CT. The information from the craniofacial region are obtained at higher resolutions at axial plane compared to CT systems . In dentistry, there are many studies showing that cone beam CT (CBCT) is widely used in the placement of implants, grafting, orthodontic treatment planning, evaluating the temporomandibular joint, detecting anatomic variations, evaluating trauma patients, caries detection .

In a study, the detection of carious lesions beneath three different ceramic restorations (zirconia, lithium disilicate, metal supported ceramic) with CBCT was investigated. It was found that the lesions of ICDAS grade 3 and above can be detected by CBCT .

Typically, the sensitivities were higher for the CBCT modalities but specificities were less, suggesting that CBCT imaging may result in an increase in the number of false-positives. Also, CBCT doses for caries detection are still higher for many types of intraoral examinations. The application of CBCT imaging to caries diagnosis is promising but more studies are needed, especially in vivo investigations. In addition, with current technology, it is assumed that teeth with metal or radiopaque restorations should not be considered for CBCT caries imaging. Another disadvantage of CBCT imaging is its high cost .

It is a new application of CT where absorbed doses and the costs are significantly lower than CT. The information from the craniofacial region are obtained at higher resolutions at axial plane compared to CT systems . In dentistry, cone beam CT (CBCT) is widely used in the placement of implants, grafting, orthodontic treatment planning, evaluating the temporomandibular joint, detecting anatomic variations, evaluating trauma patients, caries detection .

In a study for the detection of carious lesions beneath three different ceramic restorations (zirconia, lithium disilicate, metal supported ceramic) it was found that the lesions of ICDAS grade 3 and above can be detected by CBCT .

The application of CBCT imaging to caries diagnosis is promising but more studies are needed, especially in vivo investigations.

Disadvantage:

Teeth with metal or radiopaque restorations should not be considered for CBCT caries imaging. And its highly costly.

Valizadeh S, Tavakkoli MA, Karimi Vasigh H, Azizi Z, Zarrabian T. in 2012 assessed the accuracy of CBCT modality in detecting proximal carious lesions as compared to conventional periapical radiographs.[34] A diagnostic study was carried out on 84 human extracted molars and premolars. The teeth were mounted and divided in 28 blocks of 3 teeth. Periapical and CBCT images of teeth were obtained. Five observers scored the images for the detection of proximal carious lesions using a 2-point scale (caries, present; caries, absent). The gold standard was determined by histopathologic sections. Sensitivity, specificity, PPV, NPV and receiver operating charac-teristics (ROC) curves were traced for observers in both systems. The results were analyzed by paired t-test. The area under the ROC curve, sensitivity, specificity, accuracy, positive and negative predictive values of CBCT images were 0.568, 0.835, 0.637, 0.714, 0.598 and 0.856, respectively. These parameters were 0.432, 0.837, 0.722, 0.77, 0.687 and 0.858 for the periapical conventional technique, respectively.The study concluded that CBCT images did not enhance detection of proximal caries in comparison with periapical images.

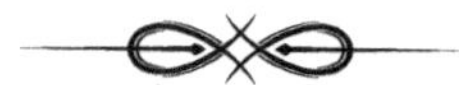

X-Ray Microtomography

X-Ray Microtomography X-ray microtomography is a shortened version of computerized axial tomography with a resolution of the order of micrometers. Microtomography (commonly known as Industrial CT scanning), like tomography, uses X-rays to create cross-sections of a 3D-object that later can be used to recreate a virtual model without destroying the original model. The term micro is used to indicate that the pixel sizes of the cross-sections are in the micrometer range.

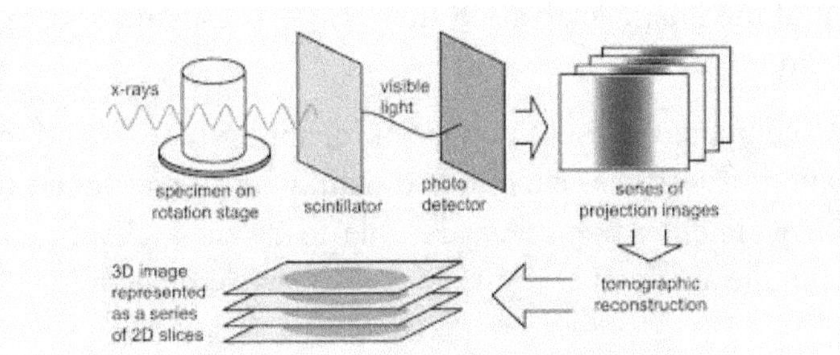

Figure 27: X Ray Microtomography

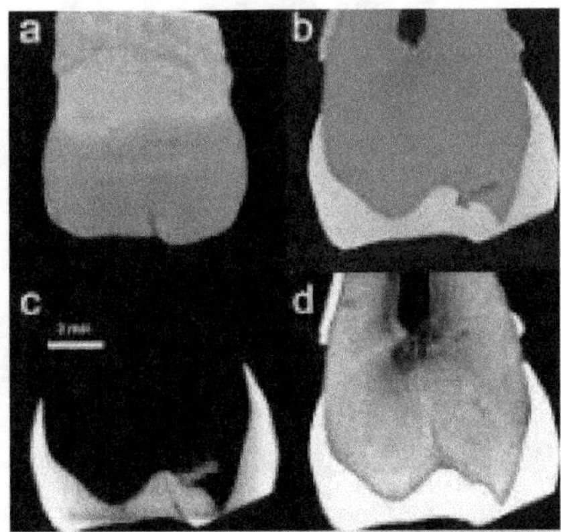

Figure 28: X Ray Microtomography

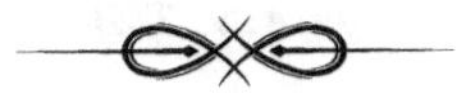

73

Transverse Microradiography (TMR)

TMR or contact-microradiography is the most practical and widely accepted method used to assess demineralization and remineralization of dental hard tissues.

Hall *et al* aimed to demonstrate the quantitative nature of LF, by means of TMR and demonstrated that LF can detect mineral loss, and, with the refinement of the image analysis system, LF was capable of detecting re-mineralization.[35]

Lo *et al.* compared the detection of changes before and after re-mineralization of artificial enamel and dentin caries and found that both micro-CT and microradiography are able to detect a change of similar magnitude in the artificial caries lesions after re- mineralization.[36]

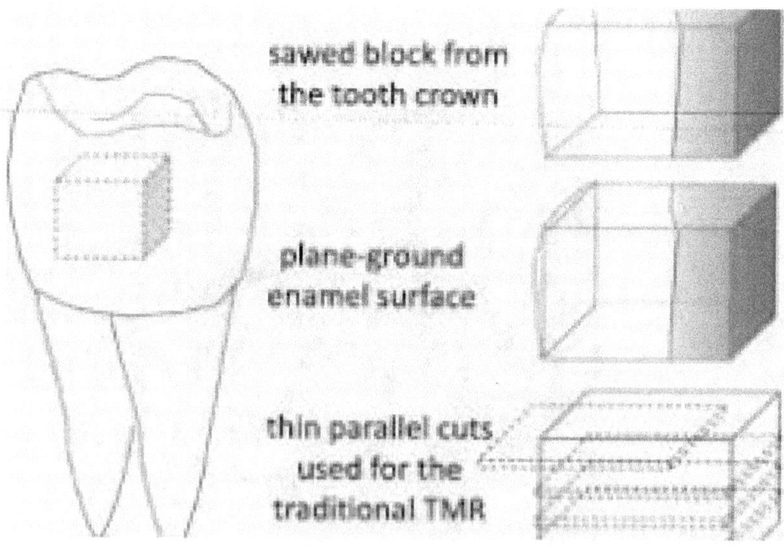

Figure 29: TMR

Tuned Aperture Ct (TACT)

TACT is a new imaging device which enhances the image by decreasing the superimposition of anatomical structures. It uses digital radiographic images and its software correlates these images into layers so that sliced sections can be viewed. A series of eight radiographs can be assimilated into one TACT image.

The use of Tuned Aperture Computed Tomography (TACT)images makes it possible to view three-dimensionalobjects in tomosynthetic radiographs.

When using TACT imaging, the degree of angular disparity between the most extreme positions of the X-ray beam needs to be adjusted for different diagnostic since it determines the `thickness' of the image layer. It has been reported that an angular disparity of158 or more should be used when maximal depth discrimination is needed

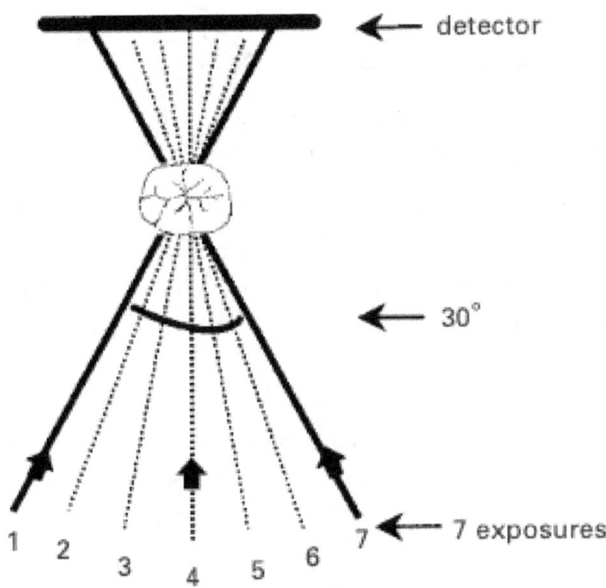

Figure 30: Diagram showing the imaging geometry for TACT .Seven exposures were obtained at 158 intervals between -15 To +15.

TACT is a new imaging device which enhances the image by decreasing the superimposition of anatomical structures. It uses digital radiographic images and its software correlates these images into layers so that sliced sections can be viewed. A series of eight radiographs can be assimilated into one TACT image.

Shi *et al.* evaluated the use of TACT for the detection of primary occlusal caries and reported that TACT radiographs were significantly better than conventional radiographs for diagnosing all types of occlusal caries. The aim of this study were to compare the difference in the accuracy of proximal caries detection by extraoral tuned aperture computed tomography (TACT), intraoral TACT, and film radiographs.

Eighty proximal surfaces of 40 extracted human maxillary teeth were used. A digital sensor was the image receptor for TACT. Film radiographs were acquired using Insight film. Nine basis images were acquired to reconstruct TACT slices. Seven observers scored the presence or absence of proximal caries using the 3 imaging modalities. The true presence of caries and its depth were determined using the sectional images obtained by micro CT. Among the image modalities and observers, possible differences in the area under the receiver operating characteristic curve were assessed by analysis of variance (ANOVA).

Results showed ANOVA indicated no statistically significant differences between observers , modalities , and observer-modality combinations .

The study concluded within the limited range of this study, extraoral TACT was not statistically different from intraoral TACT or film radiographs for proximal caries detection. This suggests that extraoral TACT may have some clinical utility for caries diagnosis and that further study may be warranted.

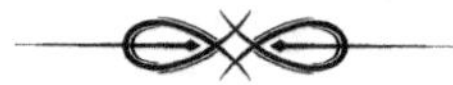

Illumination Methods

1. Fiber-Optic Transillumination (FOTI)
2. Wavelength Dependent FOTI
3. Digital Imaging Foti (DIFOTI).

FOTI (Fiber Optic Transillumination)

FOTI was initially designed by **Friedman** and **Marcus** in 1970 for the detection of proximal caries. It has higher sensitivity for dentin lesions than for enamel lesions.

Posterior approximal caries is diagnosed by placing the light probe on the gingiva below the cervical margin of the tooth, whereby light passes through the tooth structures and approximal decay appears as dark shadow on the occlusal surface. The light transmission index of decayed and sound tooth are different where sound enamel is formed of densely packed hydroxyapatite crystals. When this structure is disrupted, in the presence of demineralization, the photons of light are scattered resulting in an optical disruption . Carious tissues with fiber optic device are visible if one observes dark shadows along the dentinal tubules as it has lower light transmission index compared with the sound tooth structure . The best utilization of the **Fiber optic transillumination (FOTI)** device is for evaluating the depth of occlusal lesions (if the caries has reached to the dentin or not) and for the detection of the proximal lesions . **Fiber Optics (Optical Fiber)** refers to flexible, thin cylindrical fibers of high-optical-quality glass or plastic. The theory of fiber optics is based on SNELLS LAW which states a single optical fiber that consists of glass or plastic material with an outer cladding of a lower index of refraction material. As fiber core has a higher refractive index, light rays are reflected back into the core. The whole phenomenon is based on Snell's Law and is called **Total Internal Reflection (TIR).**

Individual fibers are grouped together to form a fiber optic bundle where fibers can be as small as 0.01 mm in diameter for glass and 0.1 mm for plastic. Fiber optics have been used in dentistry for adjunctive illumination of other devices such as handpieces and ultrasonic scalers, as well as attached to magnifying loupes.

FOTI has been a valid indicator of the histological presence or absence of bacterially infected tooth structure, with a specificity and sensitivity equivalent to or better than radiographs.

The sensitivity of a test— the true positive rate—is the percentage of people identified as having the condition. Specificity measures the proportion of negatives, ie, the percentage of individuals who do not have the condition

Techniques for Using FOTI for Tooth Evaluation

Use of the brightest light has been associated with providing the best diagnostic tool to illuminate the oral cavity and teeth and dentists use curing lights to transilluminate teeth, which recent research has demonstrated to pose a significant risk associated with "blue light hazard" that can cause retinal injury and macular degeneration and thus care should be taken while using it.

It is recommended that specialized light sources with small apertures of 3 mm or less be used, as these provide a point source that results in a sharper image for improved visualization. These smaller light guides provide white light that can be used as an indirect light for **FOTI**.

Historically in Past **FOTI** devices were large boxes with light sources that required fans for cooling and tethered electrical sources. Latest generation of light-emitting diodes (LEDs) **FOTI** devices are small, compact, and powered by batteries. The technique of moving the light angulation to change the irradiance provides a more accurate portrayal of different tooth conditions.

Principle :

FOTI works due to differences in normal enamel and dentin light transmission compared with caries, calculus, restorative materials, and external tooth discolorations.

Caries, which appears shadowed within the tooth has a lower index of light transmission than sound tooth structure. Calculus shows up as a darkened area on the surface of the tooth.

Translucent tooth- coloured restorative materials can be easily distinguished from normal tooth structure using FOTI.

Evaluating Anterior Caries

For both maxillary and mandibular anterior teeth, in order to visualize anterior proximal caries the probe should be placed on the labio-cervical region of the tooth, and the surface should be examined from the lingual aspect with a mouth mirror . In some cases, because of the thinness of mandibular incisors the light guide can be placed on the lingual surface.

Evaluating Posterior Interproximal Caries

To visualize posterior proximal caries using a conventional light guide probe is placed on the cervical area of the tooth, buccally or lingually. Light passes into the cervical tooth structure and then radiates occlusally. Caries can appear as a dark shadow on the occlusal surface.

Recently an innovative thin, flexible fiber-optic tip used for evaluating interproximal posterior caries (Microlux Proximal Caries Light Guide, AdDent, .

This 0.75-mm thin light guide is also beneficial for visualizing root canal orifices within pulp chambers. For caries diagnosis, the thin light guide tip is slid into the gingival embrasure below the proximal contact under the marginal ridge. This method often shows caries with a higher definition than a conventional fiber-optic light guide.

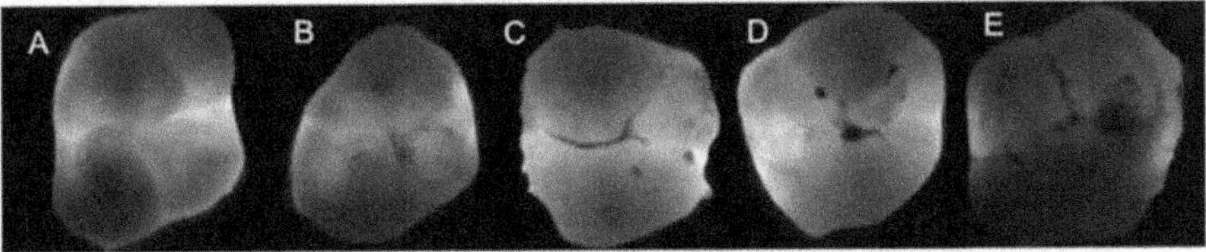

Figure 31: FOTI

Examples Of Foti Usage

FOTI can be used as a supplemental diagnostic aid for anterior and posterior interproximal caries and occlusal caries diagnosis, detection of calculus, evaluation of stained margins of composite resins, and evaluation of cusp fractures and cracked teeth.

It can also be used as an exploration tool to illuminate endodontic access and root canal orifices within the pulp chamber of teeth during endodontic treatment and as a tool for improved evaluation of soft-tissue lesions for evaluation of all-ceramic restorations to rule out any fractures before cementation, for clinical evaluation of fracture and craze lines in all-ceramic restorations and natural teeth, and for evaluation of the depth of extrinsic staining to determine appropriate treatment recommendations.

FOTI that utilizes a light emitting diode was developed for caries detection, which uses a narrow beam of white light to transilluminate the tooth. It is based on the fact that carious enamel has a lower index of light transmission than sound enamel and as the demineralization process disrupts the crystalline structure of enamel and dentin, more light is absorbed due to changes in the light scattering and absorption of light photons. In essence this gives that area a more darkened appearance.

Ie and Verdonschot conducted a Meta-analysis that showed that FOTI performed superiorly in diagnosing occlusal caries in comparison to visual inspection and xeroradiography .[37]

Ismail observed that FOTI is the most valid method for caries detection of precavitated caries in dentin followed by radiographic examination and visual examination.[38]

Peers *et al.* carried out an in vitro comparison of the performance of radiography and FOTI using histologic examination as the gold standard and they found no significant differences in the Sn values of radiography (0.59) and FOTI (0.67) with regard to approximal caries detection.[39]

FOTI is widely accepted by clinicians as a valid method for detection of approximal caries in anterior teeth as well as dentin- involved caries in posterior teeth.

Wenzel *et al.* considered transillumination to offer better performance than conventional X-rays in detecting early-stage dentin caries.

Côrtes *et al.*, conducted an in vitro study, reported greater sensitivity than specificity for FOTI and superior performance with respect to X-rays both for enamel and dentinal lesions and had a better correlation with histology.

Dental and medical transillumination refers to light transmission through tissues of the body. Majority of carious lesions are visually accessible and Caries on occlusal and buccal/lingual surfaces account for almost 90% of caries in children and adolescents. Approximately 60% of caries occur in 20% of the population, and fewer than 5% of adults are caries-free.

Caries has been identified as the single most common chronic disease of childhood and it is decreasing on interproximal surfaces, occlusal pit and fissue caries has shown a continued increase, yet the interproximal surfaces of the tooth are the least accessible to diagnose.

Accurate diagnosis of smooth-surface proximal enamel and dentin carious lesions is highly challenging to the clinician. Interproximal caries is typically diagnosed using an intraoral clinical assessment, including visualization of superficial enamel discolorations combined with using an explorer to feel for surface roughness and cavitation combined with the use of bitewing radiographs.

In most clinical cases, the access to evaluate the posterior proximal site visually and tactilely is very limited. Radiographs are an important diagnostic tool for the detection of interproximal caries,and bitewing radiographs are the most frequently used aid in assessing the potential for caries on the proximal tooth surface.

Yet, the detection of interproximal caries using bitewing radiographs has been demonstrated to have an accuracy estimated at 40% to 65%.

So ,to address the need to decrease patients' exposure to ionizing radiation, clinicians can safely evaluate difficult-to-access proximal surfaces using FOTI to supplement the clinical examination.

FOTI is a no-risk, minimally invasive, pain-free procedure that can be used repeatedly during routine dental examinations. Using a narrow beam of bright white light directed across the facial and interproximal surfaces, the dry tooth can be visualized for changes in color, texture, tooth surface appearance, and the presence or absence of shadows within the tooth.

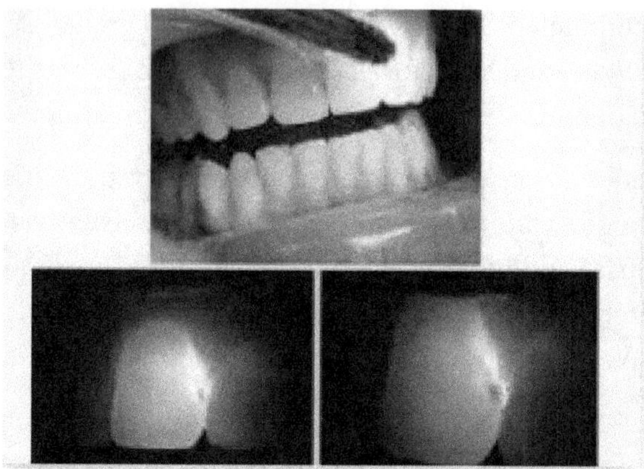

Figure 32: Detection Of Proximal Lesions By FOTI

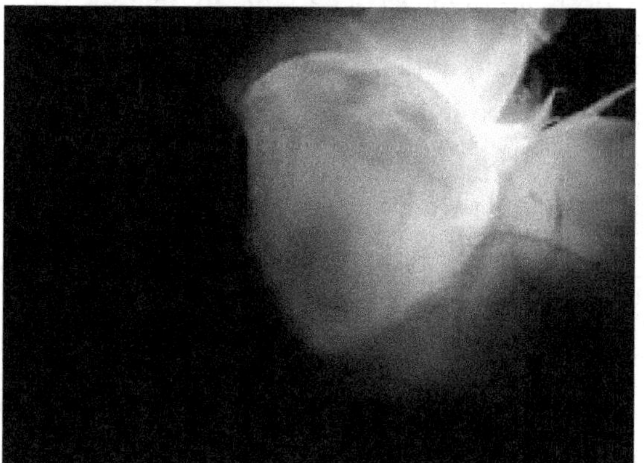

Figure 33: FOTI For Detection Of Dental Caries

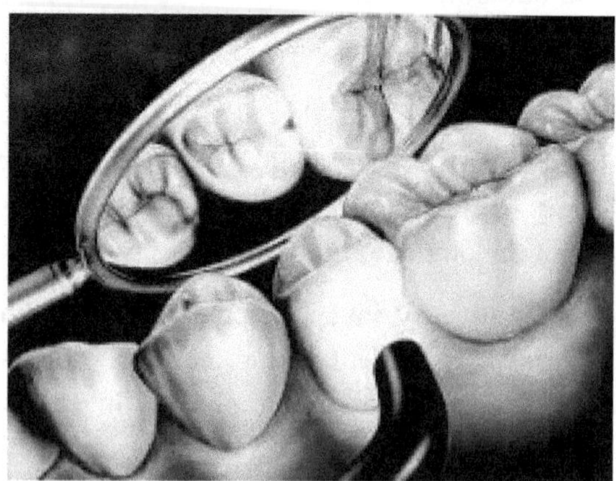

Figure 34: FOTI For Detection Of Caries

Concluding FOTI is not routinely used by dental professionals and is not recommended as a technique of choice, due to a large proportion of false-negative results. The main advantage of FOTI is its optimum positive predictive value performance, which means that any positive reading is almost certainly indicative of an existing lesion, no exposure to radiation, gives instant images simple, non time consuming, and comfortable to patients.

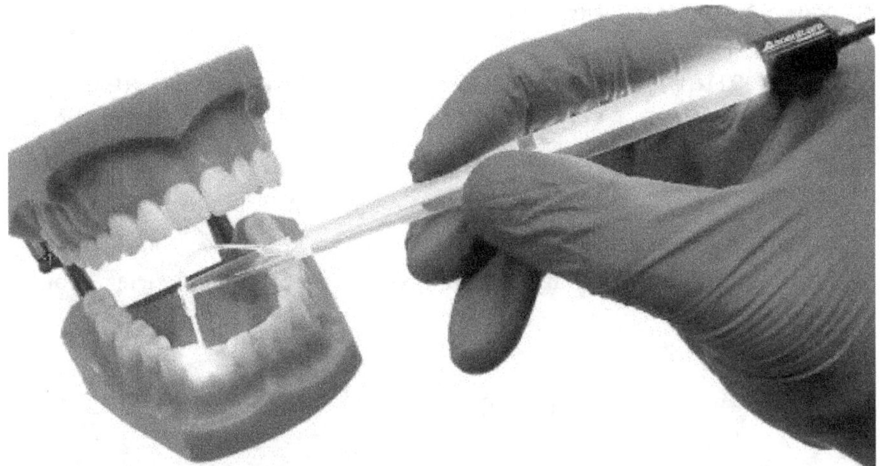

Figure 35: FOTI For Detecting Carious Lesions

Wavelength Dependent Foti

In incipient white-spot lesions, mineral loss is accompanied by an increase in light scattering. In older, discolored lesions, light absorption is also enhanced. The induced effect at the occlusal surface is caused by a combination of material properties and the distance light propagates through tooth material from the light source to the detector. This combination will be called "effective decadic optical thickness" and is dependent on the light wavelength. It is assumed that, in the case of small lesions, the effective decadic optical thickness increases linearly with mineral loss.

Vaarkamp *et al.* observed that wavelength-dependent light propagation through carious tissues can be utilized for quantitative diagnosis of approximal caries lesions. Furthermore, comparisons regarding the diagnostic performance of optical technique, bitewing radiography and dyes was performed on 33 extracted premolar teeth and it was concluded that the optical technique performed as well as bitewing radiography in diagnosing small approximal caries lesions.[40]

It has certain advantages like; it gives quantitative information about the depth of the lesion and there is no radiation hazard. However, it is not applicable in all locations of carious lesions and has considerable intra and inter-examiner variations. Based on the research, quantitative diagnosis of approximal caries lesions is feasible when wavelength-dependent light propagation through carious tissues is utilized.

Difoti Digital Fiber Optic Transillumination Imaging:

This technique was introduced to overcome the limitations of FOTI by combining FOTI and a digital charge-coupled device (CCD) camera. DIFOTI is the only dental diagnostic imaging instrument of its kind to be approved for the detection of incipient, frank, and recurrent caries. It can also be used to detect fractures, cracks, and secondary caries around restorations.

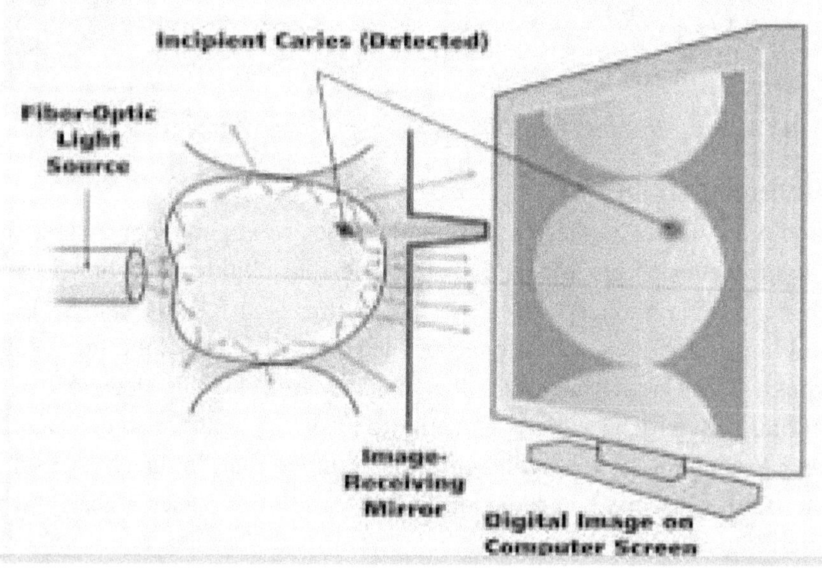

Figure 36: DIFOTI

Principle: Carious tooth tissue absorbs more light than surrounding healthy tissue and appears as darker area. DIFOTI system consists of two handpieces (one for occlusal surface and one for smooth surface and interproximal areas), a disposable mouthpiece, a foot pedal for selecting the image of interest and a computer system to capture and store the resulting image.

This method is the combination of the FOTI and a digital camera in order to reduce the shortcomings of FOTI. This system uses 780 nm wavelength near infrared radiation instead of white light source .This new detection method looks promising for identification of caries and measuring the severity of the lesions. According to studies, this method is non-invasive, doesn't use ionizing radiation and it is more sensitive than X-rays in detecting early demineralizations . It was developed in an attempt to reduce the perceived shortcomings of FOTI, by combining FOTI with a digital CCD camera. DIFOTI has elevated traditional transillumination to more sophisticated diagnostic levels

Also, the images obtained by this method can be saved and viewed later, the properties of the lesions can be examined by increasing the contrast of the image. This method is useful in detecting changes like fractures and fluorosis .

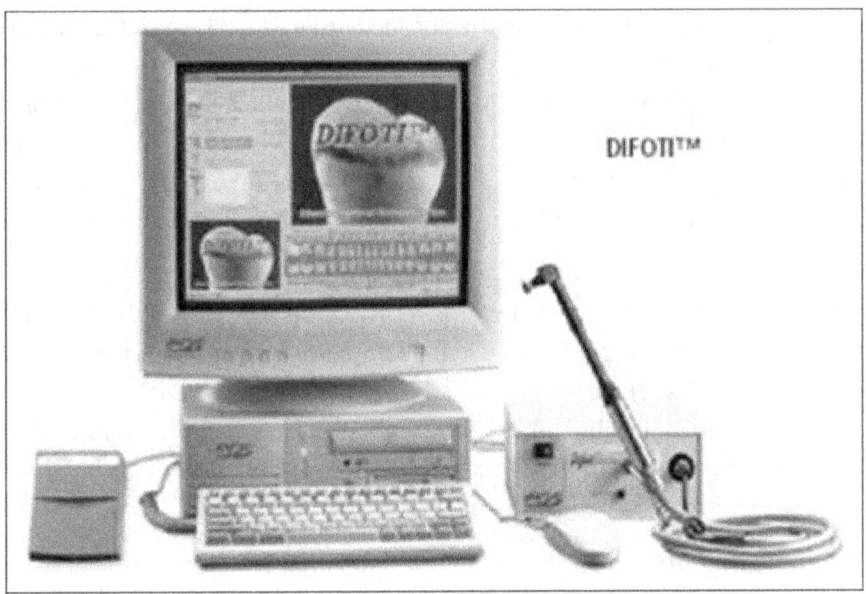

Figure 37: Digital Imaging Fiber Optic Transillumination

Mechanism Of Action

It uses a safe white light with which images taken from all the tooth surfaces can be digitally captured using a digital CCD and sent to a computer for analysis. Receptor with photocells converts photon energy to electrical energy - transmitted to a video processor and converted into color value and displayed on video monitor.

When the teeth are transilluminated, areas of demineralized enamel or dentin scatter light and incipient caries appear darker in the resultant image. Images taken during different examinations can be compared for clinical changes between several images of the same tooth over time.

Schneiderman *et al.* found that DIFOTI technique has superior sensitivity over conventional radiographic methods for the detection of approximal, occlusal, and smooth surface caries. [41]

Hae-Woong *et al.* observed that the DIFOTI diagnostic system is the most accurate means of detecting occlusal, buccal, and lingual surface carious lesions, while mesial and distal proximal carious lesions were most accurately assessed using bitewing radiography.

Kazuhiro examined the clinical usefulness of DIFOTI, to detect dental caries and cracks. Image data of the tooth obtained by visible-light fiber-optic transillumination were acquired with a digital CCD camera and sent to a computer for image analysis. Then, the incorporated data are immediately projected on the monitor as an image of the tooth. As a result, DIFOTI was shown to be effective in detecting initial caries and cracks on the surface of a tooth.

Bin-Shuwaish *et al.* evaluated the correlation between DIFOTI and clinical and radiographic images in estimating the true clinical axial extension of Class II carious lesions. It was observed that DIFOTI images correlated well with clinical depth, especially for smaller lesion. It also improved the estimation of lesion size when used in conjunction with the digital sensor and D-speed images. [42]

As reported by **Astvaldottir**, though the potential for detecting lesions in dentin by DIFOTI, Film and digital radiography is similar, the diagnostic accuracy of DIFOTI in detecting early approximal enamel lesions was greater 20.

Although it has certain advantages like gives instant images that can be stored for future references, there are several limitations of DIFOTI. The method does not measure lesion depth, and a difficulty in discriminating deep fissures, stain, and actual dentin lesions.

Overdiagnosis can occur due to lower specificity when compared with conventional radiographs. Dark areas on the images can be attributed to scatter and the absorption of light as it passes through demineralized enamel and dentin or near the surface; consequently, white spots can be mistaken for cavitations.

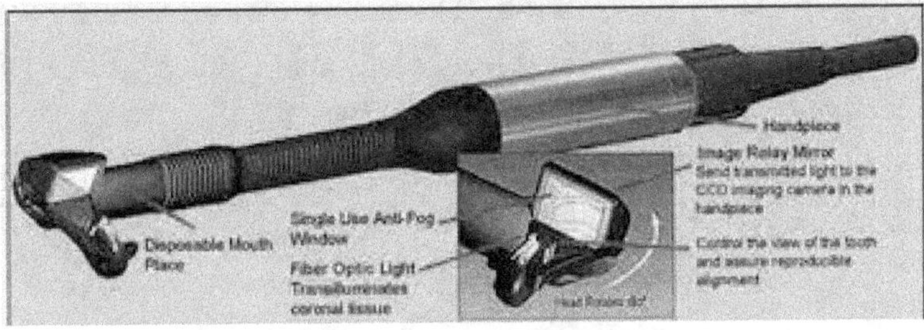

Figure 38: Apparatus DIFOTI

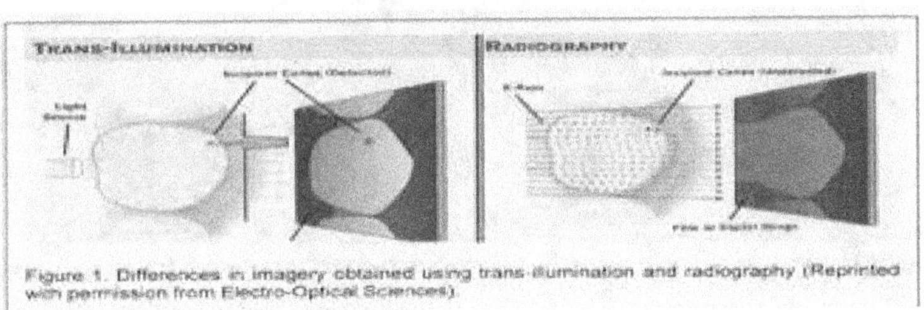

Figure 39: Differences in imagery obtained using transillumination and radiography

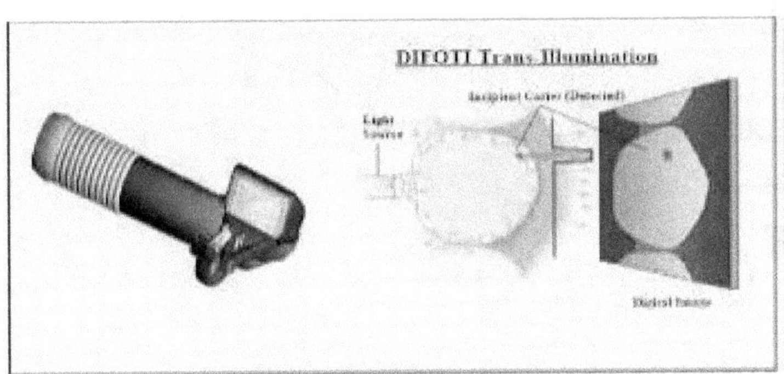

Figure 40: DIFOTI Transillumination

Mini-D

This device is based on the fiber optic principle, it is easy to use and requires no calibration. Mini-D uses LED and fiber optic technologies to detect occlusal and proximal caries lesions. This device emits 635-880 nm wavelength LED light, analyzes the light reflected from the surface of the tooth and converts it to electrical signals. The presence of caries is identified by two signals; sound and light (green light turns to red). It is also effective in wet environment but the plaque must be removed before the examination .

MIDWEST CARIES ID™ (MID)

MID is a small, battery-operated technology that emits a soft LED light for detecting and quantifying caries. A specific fiber optic signature captures the resulting reflection and refraction of the light in the tooth and is converted to electrical signals that run through a computer-based algorithm for analyzing the presence of caries.

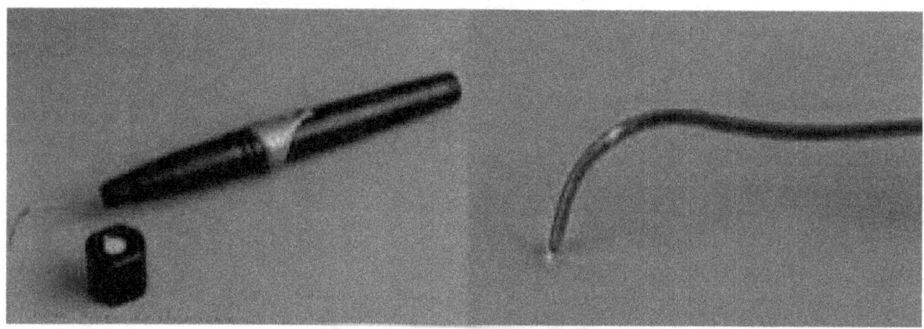

Figure 41: Midwest Caries ID

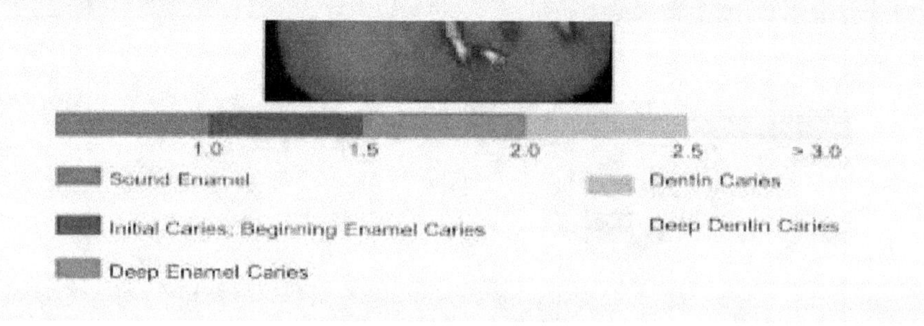

Figure 42: Colour Coding

Patel *et al.* reported the sensitivity and specificity for this detection device as 0.56 and 0.84, respectively.

Krause *et al.* reported sensitivity of 100%, which was calculated by comparing the Midwest to radiographic findings.[43]

Rodrigues *et al.* assessed the performance of two LED (MID and Vista Proof-VP) and two laser fluorescence (LF)- based devices (DIAGNOdent 2095-LF and DIAGNOdent pen 2190-LF pen) in detecting occlusal caries in vitro on 97 permanent molars. Both LF devices seem to be useful as supplementary tools to conventional methods, presenting good reproducibility and better accuracy. Furthermore, MID could not differentiate sound surfaces from enamel caries and VP still needs perfection on the cutoff limits for its use.

Aktan *et al.* compared laser-based (DIAGNOdent) and LED-based (MID) in the detection of occlusal caries and concluded that MID device more regularly revealed the presence of occlusal caries in comparison to DIAGNOdent pen.

Van Hilsen and Jones evaluated and compared MID, visual photographic examination (CAM) and cross- polarization optical coherence tomography (CP-OCT) observed that MID and CP-OCT were useful in detecting the presence of demineralization, but cannot be utilized to adequately assess the depth of the demineralization.

LED technology (Midwest Caries I.D.): Recently, a device based on LED technology – Midwest Caries I.D. – (DENTSPLY Professional, York, PA, USA) is developed for caries detection. The handheld device emits a soft light emitting diode (LED) between 635 nm and 880 nm and analyzes the reflectance and refraction of the emitted light from the tooth surface, which is captured by fiber optics and is converted to electrical signals for analysis. The microprocessor of the device contains a computer-based algorithm that identifies the different optical signature (changes in optical translucency and opacity) between healthy and demineralized tooth.

Endoscopy

Endoscopy includes:

- Endoscopically viewed filtered fluorescence
- White light fluorescence
- Videoscope.

Endoscopically viewed filtered fluorescence

This technique utilizes the fluorescence of enamel that occurs when it is illuminated with blue light in wavelength range 499–500 nm. When the tooth is viewed from a specific gelatine green filter number 58, attached to the eyepiece, white spot lesions appear darker than sound enamel.

Pitts and Longbottom explored the use of EFF for the clinical diagnosis of carious lesions and compared results with conventional alternatives on occlusal and approximal sites. The EFF method has been shown to be highly sensitive for occlusal enamel caries and high specificity for approximal lesions at both thresholds. This work developed to include the use of an intraoral video system for caries detection, the prototype "videoscope."

Longbottom and Pitts compared the diagnostic performance of visual endoscopic caries diagnosis (with and without the benefit of differential fluorescence) with that of conventional visual diagnosis, bitewing radiography, and conventional transillumination. The study concluded that endoscopic methods detected a greater number of carious lesions than do conventional visual, radiographic, or FOTI methods.

Advantage :

It gives a magnified view of carious lesions and provides large range of viewing angles, and the areas, which are difficult to view by conventional means, are easily accessible. However, it has few limitations like being time consuming and technique sensitive. Thus meticulous drying and isolation are necessary for accurate results.

White light fluorescence

A white light source is connected to the endoscope by a fiber- optic cable and teeth are viewed without a filter. It has certain limitations like weight of fiber-optic cable tends to destabilize the machine and the increased distance between eyepiece and light source decreases illumination.

Videoscope

The integration of the camera and endoscope is called a videoscope. This is designed in such a way that the image of the surface of enamel can be viewed directly over a television screen. The videotapes are viewed by expert independent examiners who had also examined the teeth visually and by conventional methods.

It has certain advantages like providing a magnified image and being clinically feasible. However, it requires meticulous drying and isolation of teeth and is time consuming and very costly thus making it for limited use only.

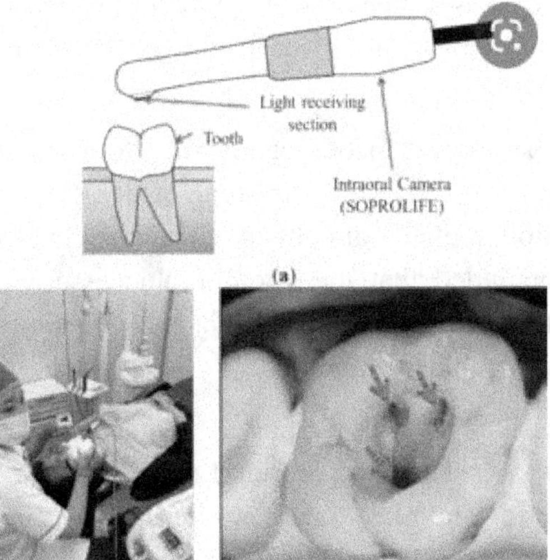

Figure 43: Soprolife

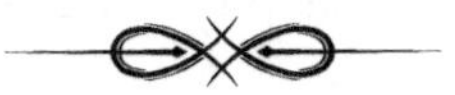

Intraoral Television Camera (IOTV)

It is based on the same idea as endoscopes, using a small visualization device to provide a better view of the oral cavity. The intraoral wand camera projects magnified digital images from a patient's mouth. Through the IOTV, the dentist can educate the patient and at the same time, can also improve their own diagnostic expertise as they see magnified oral conditions which are significantly better than direct vision.

Advantages:

increased vision,

improved posture, and patient positioning, and

increased magnification

Forgie *et al.* concluded that IOVC can achieve very high level of sensitivity, but this is accompanied with drop in specificity and not suitable for large epidemiological surveys which require extensive human and economic resources.

Boye *et al.* compared diagnostic performance for the detection of caries using photographs (taken with intra-oral camera) with an established visual examination method and histological sections as the reference standard and concluded that the photographic assessment method had higher sensitivity for caries detection than visual examination. The two methods had comparable specificities.

Paul *et al.* described a laser-supported dental endoscope, which is a combination of a customary intraoral camera with a laser as an illumination source. The use of a laser beam at 530 nm for illumination enables a significant presentation of early caries on tooth enamel. The laser-supported dental endoscope, employing a laser beam of 337 nm, is also suitable to detect early caries on the basis of the autofluorescence of the tooth enamel.

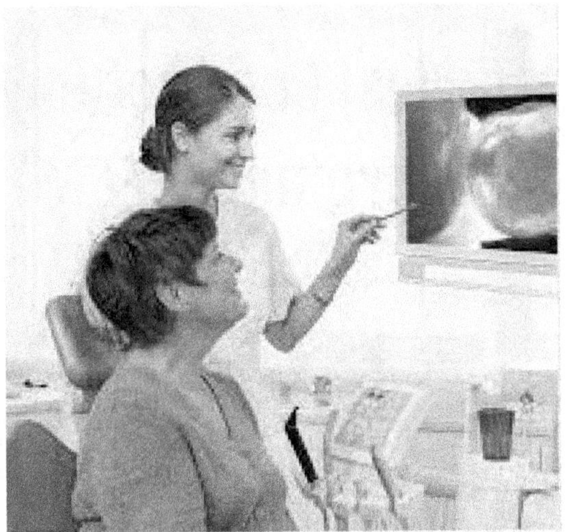

Figuure 44: Intraoral Camera

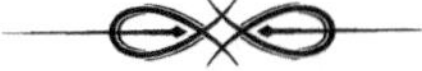

Electrical Conductance Measurement (ECM)

The idea of an electrical method for caries detection was proposed by **Magitot** in 1878, and is based on the theory that sound dental hard tissue, especially the enamel, shows very high electrical resistance or impedance. In the impedance measurement system a circuit of a very weak alternating current is closed through the patient. From the device, a fiber leads to a probe, which is placed on the site that is to be measured.

Based on the differences in the electrical conductance of carious tissue and sound enamel, two instruments were developed and tested in 1980, i.e. **Vanguard electronic caries detector** and **Caries Meter.**[44]

In Vanguard electronic caries detector method, resistance measurements are made between a hand held connection and probe tip placed within the fissures of the teeth. Superficial saliva is removed to prevent surface conduction. Machine gives a reading on a scale of 0-9, which is directly proportional to the degree of demineralization. Vangaurd electronic caries detectormanufactured by Massachusetts Manufacturing Corp., Cambridge, Mass, USA. Electrical conductivity is expressed numerically on a scale from 0 to 9. The machine displayed a frowning face that indicated extensive demineralization or the smiling face that indicated a sound site. This device is no longer available commercially

In Caries Meter method, the resistance measurement is made between the probe tip and clip attached to oral electrode, and coloured light reflects the status of tooth.

Advantages: Small and handy systems, accurate diagnosis and no pain to the patient.

Disadvantages: are that the area of diagnosis is confined to the dimension of the probe, technique sensitivity as salivary or temperature changes can change measurements and the status of lesion is not known such as arrested or active.

Principle :

A demineralized tooth has more pores filled with water or saliva, and this is more conductive than intact tooth surface.

Greater the amount of demineralization, higher is the electrical conductivity through enamel. Demineralized sites and sites with high pore volume and cavities can be detected by measuring the conductance.

This technique has two methods of application.

a) Site-specific

Applies probe as electrode into fissures and the electrical conductance of that site is measured. To prevent current from leaking through superficial layer of moisture through the gingival, airflow is applied to dry the tooth surface around the probe. Disadvantage is that only small areas of occlusal surface can be measured at one time

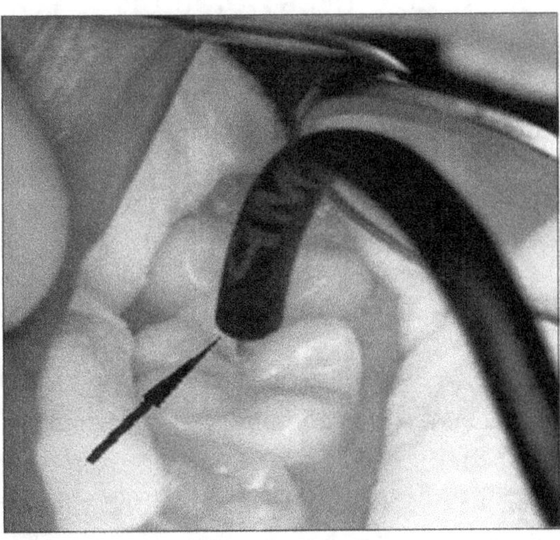

Figure 45: Site Specific

b)Surface-Specific

This technique measures the entire occlusal surface, which is covered with an electrolyte-containing medium where the electrode is placed. ECM uses a fixed frequency of 23 Hz alternate current

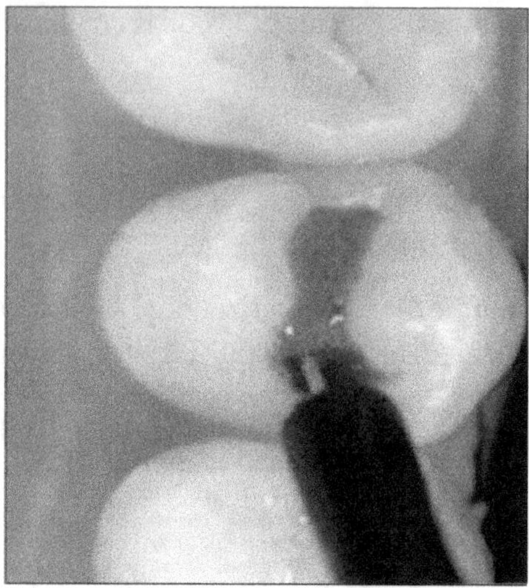

Figure 46: ECM

Two instruments based on the difference in electrical conductance of carious and sound enamel were developed.

Vanguard Electronic Caries Detector

It used a current of 25 Hz. Measured conductance was then converted to an ordinary scale of 0-9. Moisture and saliva were removed by a continuous stream of air to prevent surface conductance.

Electronic Caries Monitor (ECM) –

The device employs a single, fixed-frequency alternating current which attempts to measure the 'bulk resistance' of tooth tissue This can be undertaken at either a site or surface level. When measuring the electrical properties of a particular site on a tooth, the ECM probe is directly applied to the site, typically a fissure, and the site measured. During the 5 s measurement cycle, compressed air is expressed from the tip of the probe and this results in a collection of data over the measurement period, described as a drying profile that can provide useful information for characterizing the lesion. It is generally accepted that the increase in porosity associated with caries is responsible for the mechanism of action for ECM, There are number of physical factors that will affect ECM results. These include the temperature of the tooth, the thickness of the tissue, the hydration of the material (i.e. one should not dry the teeth prior to use) and the surface area.

The idea of an electrical method for caries detection was proposed by Magitot in 1878, and is based on the theory that sound dental hard tissue, especially the enamel, shows very high electrical resistance or impedance. In the impedance measurement system a circuit of a very weak alternating current is closed through the patient. From the device, a fiber leads to a probe, which is placed on the site that is to be measured.

Based on the differences in the electrical conductance of carious tissue and sound enamel, two instruments were developed and tested in 1980, i.e. Vanguard electronic caries detector and caries meter. In Vanguard electronic caries detector method, resistance measurements are made between a hand held connection and probe tip placed within the fissures of the teeth. Superficial saliva is removed to prevent surface conduction. Machine gives a reading on a scale of 0-9, which is directly proportional to the degree of demineralization. In caries meter method, the resistance measurement is made between the probe tip and clip attached to oral electrode, and colored light reflects the status of tooth.

Disadvantages:

The area of diagnosis is confined to the dimension of the probe,

Technique sensitivity as salivary or temperature changes can change measurements

Status of lesion is not known such as arrested or active.

Advantages are small and handy systems, accurate diagnosis and no pain to the patient. Sengun *et al.* found that the ECM is very useful at the diagnosis of occlusal caries which are difficult to detect clinically and in this way minimizes the risk of unnecessary tissue loss. With this device, it can be possible to avoid unnecessary radiographs.

Various studies have shown that ECM has higher sensitivity values (0.90) compared with conventional methods for detecting occlusal dentin caries lesions. However, lower specificity values (around 0.80) have been observed. In Ashley *et al.* study, surface-specific electrical measurements were recorded every 6 months during the second 18-month period of a 3-

year clinical trial comparing two products whose relative anti-caries effects were unknown. Over an 18-month period, ECM measurements demonstrated a significant difference in the mean distributed file system increment between the test and the control groups. In contrast, the conventional detection methods used in the trial were unable to discriminate between the products over three years.

Improved diagnoses at the dentinal level were obtained, when EC and LF were used at higher cutoff values as an adjunct to visual inspection, as the latter rely exclusively on fissure discoloration. In cases of discolored fissures, these methods help to overcome false-positive identification of dentinal caries. However, attainable reliabilities of diagnoses do not seem to exceed about 50–60%.

Fennis-Ie *et al.* compared the performance of visual inspection on FOTI, and electrical conductance measurements (ECMs) and concluded that ECM is a better predictor of occlusal caries than fissure discoloration and FOTI. A cost-effective analysis is envisaged to obtain insight into the practical value of ECMs in the prediction of occlusal caries and, thus, into the effectiveness of sealant application.

The ECM readings may range between -0.70 and 13.20 indicating increased conductance.(Fig - 05).

Interpretation Of Values

-1.00 to 3.00=sound enamel or incipient stage of caries 3.01 to 6.00=caries upto the DEJ (enamel caries)

6.01 to 8.00=dentinal caries

8.01 to 13.00=extending half of dentine thickness

Sengun *et al.* found that the ECM is very useful at the diagnosis of occlusal caries which are difficult to detect clinically and in this way minimizes the risk of unnecessary tissue loss. With this device, it can be possible to avoid unnecessary radiographs.

Various studies have shown that ECM has higher sensitivity values (0.90) compared with conventional methods for detecting occlusal dentin caries lesions. However, lower specificity values (around 0.80) have been observed.

Ashley *et al.* study, surface-specific electrical measurements were recorded every 6 months during the second 18-month period of a 3-year clinical trial comparing two products whose relative anti-caries effects were unknown. Over an 18-month period, ECM measurements demonstrated a significant difference in the mean distributed file system increment between the test and the control groups. In contrast, the conventional detection methods used in the trial were unable to discriminate between the products over three years.

Improved diagnoses at the dentinal level were obtained, when EC and LF were used at higher cut off values as an adjunct to visual inspection, as the latter rely exclusively on fissure discoloration. In cases of discolored fissures, these methods help to overcome false-positive identification of dentinal caries. However, attainable reliabilities of diagnoses do not seem to exceed about 50–60%.

Fennis-Ie *et al.* compared the performance of visual inspection on FOTI, and electrical conductance measurements (ECMs) and concluded that ECM is a better predictor of occlusal caries than fissure discoloration and FOTI. A cost-effective analysis is envisaged to obtain insight into the practical value of ECMs in the prediction of occlusal caries and, thus, into the effectiveness of sealant application.

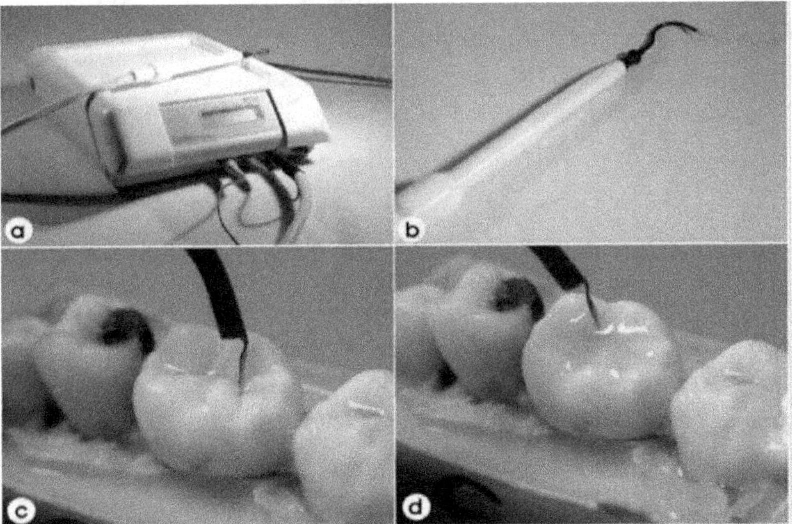

Figure 47: ECM

Impedence values		
Colour	Impedance value	Indication
Green	600 KΩ	Healthy tooth
Yellow	Between 250 & 600 KΩ	Enamel caries
Orange	Between 15 & 250 KΩ	Caries extending into dentin
Red	Below 15 KΩ	Caries reaching to tooth pulp exposed to bacterial infection.

Figure 48: Impedence Values

Fluorescence

Two methods have been developed based on the fluorescence of the organic components of teeth; they are quantitative light-induced fluorescence [QLF (QLF-clin, Inspector Research Systems BV, Amsterdam, Netherlands)] which uses an arc lamp with a wavelength of 290-450 nm and DIAGNOdent (KaVo Dental laser fluorescence pen, DIAGNOdent pen, Lake Zurich) which uses infrared light and has a 655 nm wavelength .

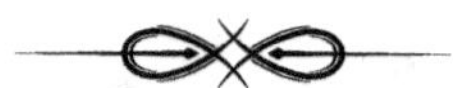

Diagnodent – Laser Autofluorescence

DIAGNOdent was first introduced in 1998 to aid the diagnosis of occlusal caries in adjunct to visual and radiographic examination. It is a variant of QLF system and was introduced based on research by Hibst and Gal. [45]

DIAGNOcam was proposed to the market with the technology which uses a laser diode of wavelength 780 nm for transillumination of teeth. Carious tissues absorb lighter than their surroundings and a digital camera is used for monitoring the images. The caries tissues appear as dark spots.Results obtained by DIAGNO cam were better correlating with the clinical results when compared with DIAGNOdent . Another new technology is DIAGNOdent pen (KaVo Dental, Biberach, Germany). This device works with the same principle as DIAGNOdent and it comes with two different sapphire fiber tips: A cylindrical tip and a conical tip. In a study comparing DIAGNOdent and DIAGNOdent pen in detecting occlusal caries it was found that this new device gives comparable results with DIAGNOdent

This system has a range of 0 to 99. The value 0 indicates the healthiest state of the tooth and is an effective method in detecting initial lesions without cavitation. It's also useful for measuring different decalcification values in different surfaces of the tooth. The fiber optic probe directed onto the occlusal surface of the tooth emits a light of wavelength 655 nm. The changes caused by demineralization are converted into numeric values and displayed on the screen. The surface to be examined must be clean because dental calculus, plaque and discoloration may cause false results.

DIAGNOdent has high sensitivity for caries detection and low specifity means a higher rate of false positive results are obtained. Therefore, it is recommended to use DIAGNOdent in combination with other techniques . It is a laser diode generates a pulsed 655 nm laser beam through a central fiber, which is transported to the tip of the device and into the tooth. When the incident light interacts with tooth substance, it stimulates fluorescent (or luminescent) light at longer wavelengths. The intensity of fluorescence depends on the degree of demineralization or bacterial concentration in the probed region.

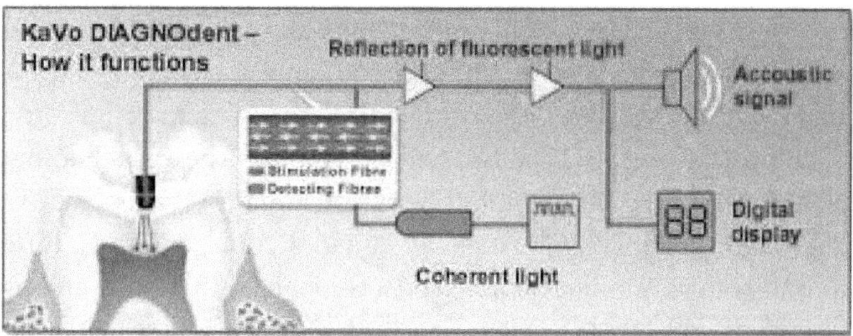

Figure 49: Diagnodent Scale

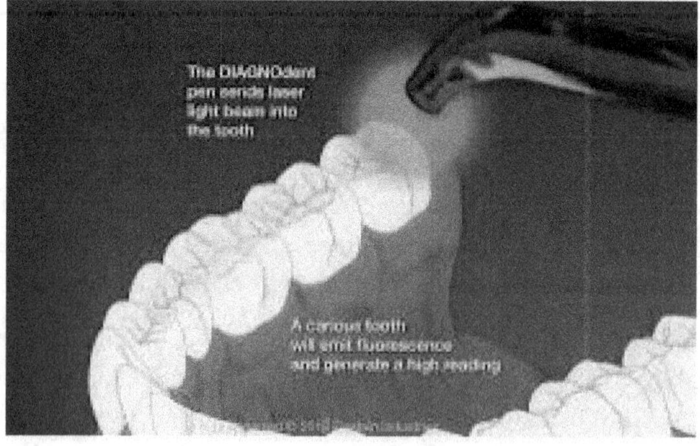

Figure 50: Function Of Diagnodent

Figure 51: Diagnodent

Diagnodent include 90% success rate in diagnosing pit and fissure caries, higher sensitivity (0.92) than electronic caries monitor, high reproducibility and reliability, easy and quick to use, readily transportable, non-invasive and painless, does not suffer from operative bias, safe, and no X-ray exposure. However, it has certain limitations like false results with the presence of plaque and debris, cannot distinguish between hypomineralized and carious structure, readings do not relate to the amount of dentinal decay, and cannot be used for recurrent caries. Shi *et al.* carried out in vitro study and concluded that the diagnostic performance of the DIAGNOdent method was superior to that of radiography.

Reis *et al.* compared the DIAGNOdent readings on three different macroscopically sound and intact occlusal surfaces and compare with visual and radiographic inspection and concluded that in a low prevalence sample, the visual inspection provided the highest proportion of true disease and DIAGNOdent provided the highest proportion of non-disease identified correctly.

Goel *et al.* concluded that DIAGNOdent showed higher sensitivity and accuracy as compared with other conventional methods (visual and tactile examination and bitewing radiographs) for detection of enamel caries, whereas for detection of dentinal caries, even though the sensitivity was high, accuracy of the DIAGNOdent device was similar to other conventional caries diagnostic methods.

Pinheiro *et al.* and Khalife *et al.* reported that, although the laser device had acceptable performance, this equipment should be used as an adjunct method to visual inspection to avoid false-positive results.

Dental laser diagnostic is a non-ionizing diagnostic method based on the measurement of the fluorescence of the enamel and dentin. Demineralized enamel has different optical attributes compared to the healthy enamel. Demineralized enamel can visually be seen as a white spot lesion. The optical change is caused by increased pore volume in the demineralized enamel. This change of the optical values can be quantified by a laser fluorescence device and theoretically it can be used to identify early caries lesions.

Armamentarium:

The LF device consists of 655 nm monochromatic light that is emitted from a tip/sensor and can detect back-scattered fluorescence from the tooth. At 655 nm, the fluorophores have been identified as bacterial porphyrins. The DD scores ranges between 0 and 99. This number offers the possibility to monitor lesion behavior. An example of such a device is the Kavo DIAGNO dent. It is a small chairside battery powered laser fluorescence device. It is used by scanning the area of interest and noting the peak value that the device shows. The value can then be interpreted to decide whether treatment is needed. The values will vary depending on age, tooth color, staining, and location of lesions. The recommended cut-off value that yields the highest sensitivity and specificity can be found in scientific literature.

The Kavo DIAGNOdent method shows a very high sensitivity for low cut-off values. Cut-off values are the baseline for which higher values will be interpreted as the presence of caries lesions. Unfortunately the specificity is poor for low values. This may be caused by calculus, fillings and/or stain that will give an artificial high value, which can be interpreted as caries.

Studies do however report excellent intra-examinator reliability and good to excellent inter examinor reliability by using the **Kavo DIAGNOdent**, i.e. getting a correct value does not seem to be affected by experience. It is a viable tool for the diagnosis of occlusal dentin caries, and studies even suggest that the KaVo DIAGNOdent combined with the visual-tactile method is a superior diagnostic option for the diagnosis of fissure caries, compared to the visual-tactile method supplemented with radiographs.

It is also a useful diagnostic tool, in combination with the visual-tactile method, for detection of proximal lesions. Accurate results have however been difficult to obtain in cases of tight contact points, due to the large tip of the tool.

A smaller tip is suggested to help aid better diagnostics. When it comes to the detection of early caries lesions, the reports are more mixed.

According to one study, the KaVo DIAGNOdent could differentiate between caries up to the EDJ and dentin caries in proximal lesions by a sensitivity of 0,6 and a specificity of 0,84 given a cut off value of 16. This implies that there is no significant difference between dental radiographs and the KaVo DIAGNOdent when it comes to the diagnosis of early proximal caries lesions in permanent teeth.

Diagnodent with a laser diode generates a pulsed 655 nm laser beam through a central fiber, which is transported to the tip of the device and into the tooth. When the incident light interacts with tooth substance, it stimulates fluorescent (or luminescent) light at longer wavelengths. The intensity of fluorescence depends on the degree of demineralization or bacterial concentration in the probed region.

Advantages:

- 90% success rate in diagnosing pit and fissure caries
- Higher sensitivity (0.92) than electronic caries monitor
- High reproducibility and reliability
- Easy and quick to use
- Readily transportable
- Non-invasive and painless
- Does not suffer from operative bias
- Safe
- No x-ray exposure.

Limitations like false results with the presence of plaque and debris, cannot distinguish between hypomineralized and carious structure, readings do not relate to the amount of dentinal decay, and cannot be used for recurrent caries.

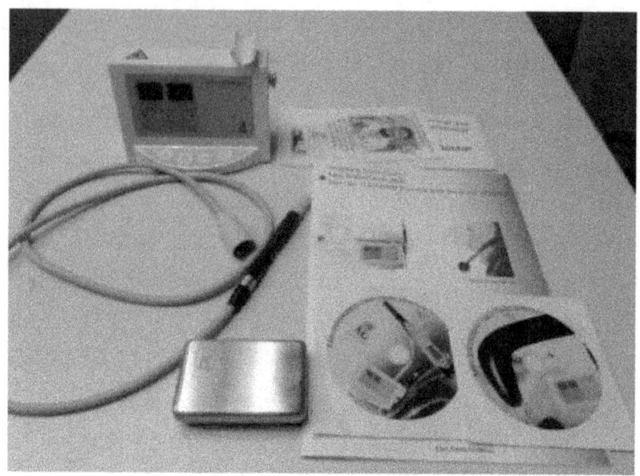

Figure 52: Kavo Diagnodent Laser Caries Detection AID

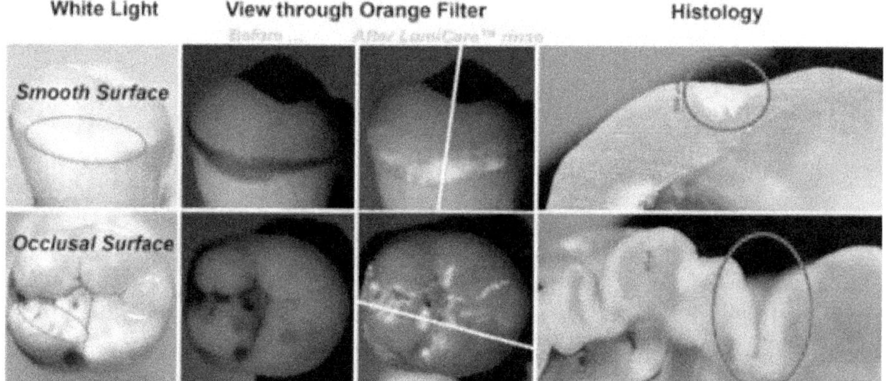

Figure 53: Detection Of Occlusal And Smooth Surface Caries

Example of the analysis of dental structures and caries tagging. The observers drew lines for the segmentation of dental structures (enamel, dentin, pulp, metal restoration, tooth-color restorations, gutta percha) and dental caries on the bitewing radiographs.

Dentist's tagging   Deep learning model

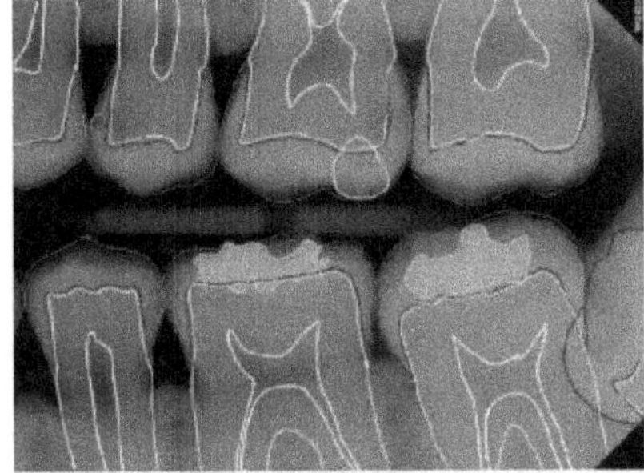 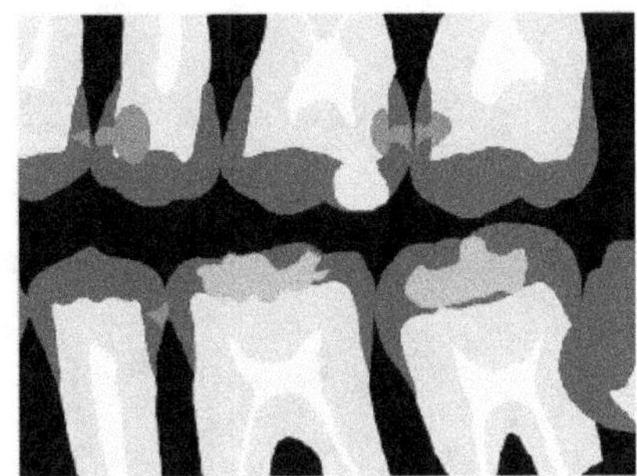

Caries (red), enamel (blue), dentin (green), pulp ( ), metal restoration (orange), restoration (sky blue), gutta percha (brown), background (black)

Figure 54: Dentist Tagging

Mechanism Of Action

DIAGNOdent technology uses a simple laser diode to compare the reflection wavelength against a well-known healthy baseline to uncover decay.

At specific wavelength that the device operates, healthy tooth structure exhibits little or no fluorescence, resulting in very low scale readings on the display. Carious tooth structure exhibits fluorescence proportionate to the degree of caries, resulting in elevated scale readings on the display. The unit has a fiber-optic cable that transmits light source to a handpiece that contains a fiber-optic eye in the tip. First, the laser diode is aimed at the healthy enamel tooth structure to obtain a benchmark reading. After calibration, it is moved to inspect all the surfaces of the teeth, shining the laser at 2.5 mm into all suspected areas.

As the laser pulses into grooves, fissures, and cracks, it reflects fluorescent light with particular wavelength. This is because light is absorbed by the organic and inorganic components of the tooth which induce infrared fluorescence.

This fluorescence is collected at the top of handpiece and transmitted back to the **DIAGNOdent unit.** Light is measured by receptors, converted into an acoustic signal, and evaluated electronically to reveal values between 0 and 9

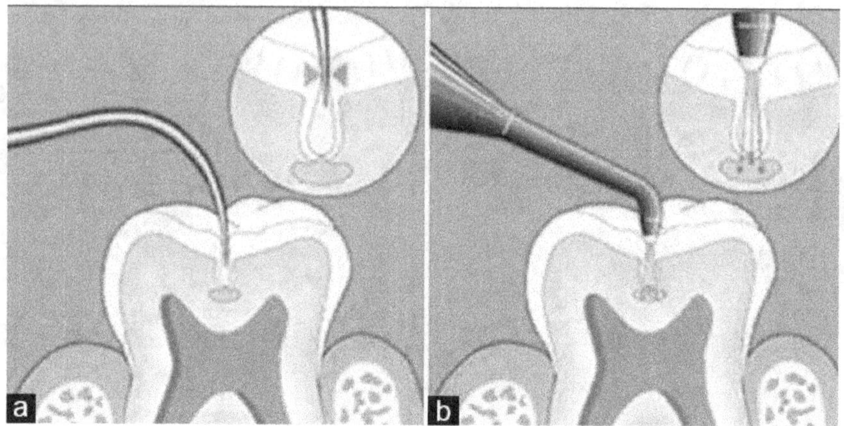

Figure 55: DIAGnodent Mechanism Of Action

Carbon Dioxide Laser

The reason of the application of carbon dioxide laser as a diagnostic tool is because the subsurface of the carious lesion has more organic compounds than the adjacent sound tissues. When carbon dioxide laser is applied to an incipient lesion, the organic contents evaporate leaving a black carbonized residue behind whereas the inorganic substance of sound enamel containing minimum amount of water is less affected by the laser beam .

More clinical studies should be carried out in order to understand the efficacy of carbon dioxide laser.

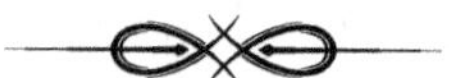

Cariescan

This device is based on alternating current impedance spectroscopy and involves the passing of an insensitive level of electrical current through the tooth to identify the presence and location of the decay. It is the first dental diagnostic tool to use an impedance spectroscopy to quantify dental caries early enough to enhance preventative treatment. CarieScan is not affected by optical factors such as staining or discoloration of the tooth.

It provides a qualitative value based on the disease state rather than the optical properties of the tooth.

Bader *et al.* carried out a systematic review comparing CarieScan with a clinical visual examination, bitewing radiograph, and DIAGNOdent reported CarieScan to have superior sensitivity and specificity both 92.5% over other methods.[46]

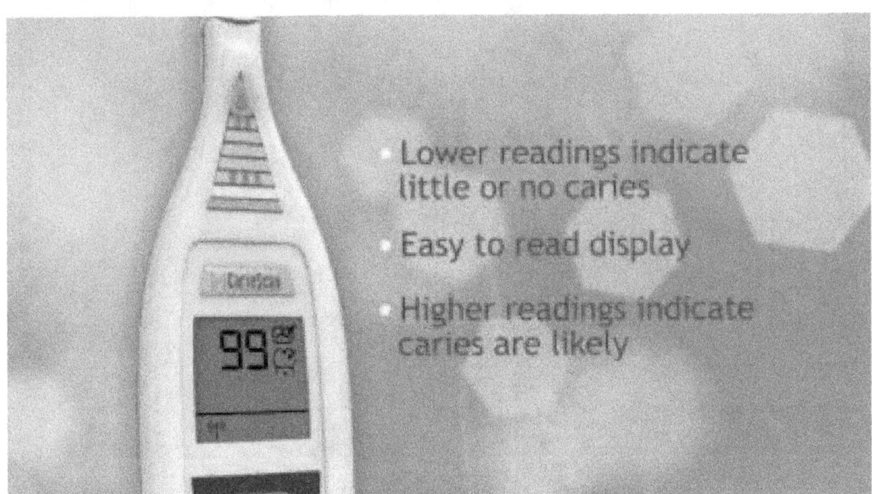

Figure 56: Cariescan

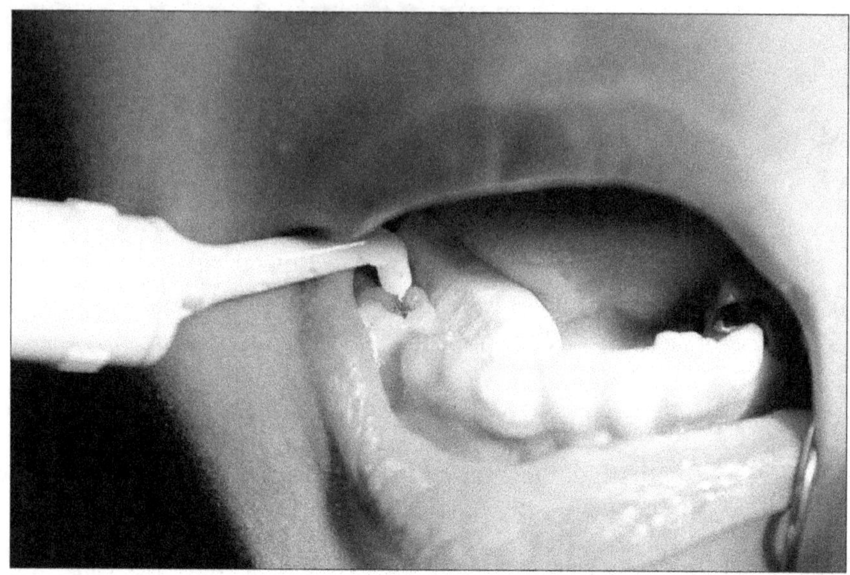

Figure 57: Cariescan

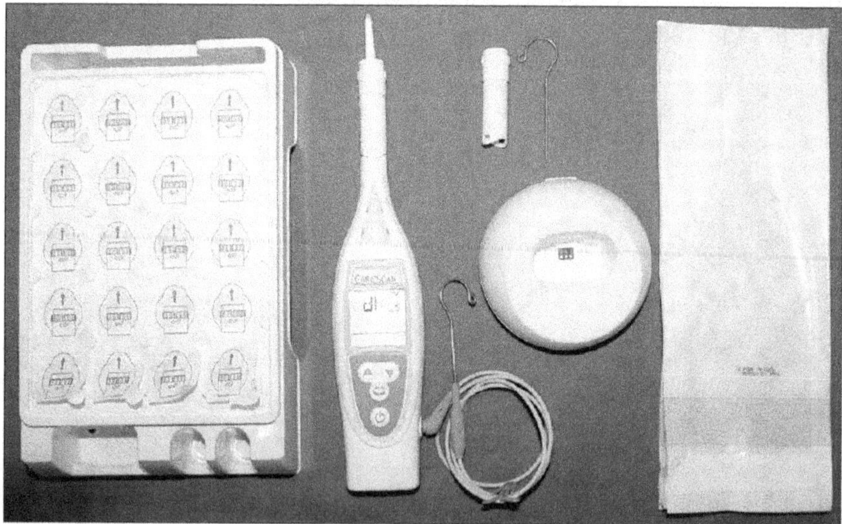

Figure 58: Armamentarium Of Cariescan

Score	Visual inspection	Bitewing radiograph	CarieScan PRO	Validation method
0	No caries	No radiolucency	0-50 (green LED[T] pyramid)	No caries
1	Caries confined to enamel	Radiolucency confined to enamel	51-90 (yellow LED[T] pyramid)	Enamel caries
2	Caries extending to dentin	Radiolucency extending to dentin	91-100 (red LED[T] pyramid)	Dentinal caries

[T]LED=Light emitting diode

Figure 59: Visual Inspection, Bitewing Radiograph , Cariescan And Validation Method

Scores for diagnosis of occlusal caries by visual inspection , bite wing radiography.

Caries scan PRO and validation method.

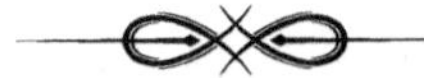

OCT

The first OCT in the field of dentistry was performed by Colston *et al.* in 1998. It creates cross-sectional images of biological structures using, differences in reflection of light. Microstructural details are revealed by differentiating between scattered, transmitted, or reflected photons.

Baumgartner *et al.* showed that it can provide additional information related to the mineralization status and/or the scattering properties of the dental materials.

Amaechi *et al.* investigated the correlation between fluorescence loss measured by QLF and the reflectivity loss measured by a OCT system in a demineralization process to produce artificial dental caries and concluded that the decrease in reflectivity of the enamel during demineralization, measured by OCT, could be related to the amount of mineral lost during the demineralization process.

Nguyen *et al.* reported that the diagnostic capability of OCT (78–88% sensitivity and 71–84% specificity) was best in superficial, inter-proximal areas, and margins of restorations and was least effective in deep caries at locations exceeding 2 mm depth and concluded that OCT is a rapidly developing, promising modality for in vivo real-time imaging with excellent capability for non-invasive early caries detection and monitoring.

Microstructural details are revealed by differentiating between scattered, transmitted, or reflected photons. Baumgartner *et al.* showed that it can provide additional information related to the mineralization status and/or the scattering properties of the dental materials.

Amaechi *et al.* investigated the correlation between fluorescence loss measured by QLF and the reflectivity loss measured by a OCT system in a demineralization process to produce artificial dental caries and concluded that the decrease in reflectivity of the enamel during demineralization, measured by OCT, could be related to the amount of mineral lost during the demineralization process.

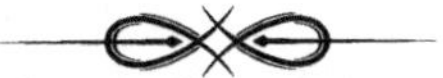

Species Specific Monoclonal Antibodies

Shi *et al.* in 1998, identified specific monoclonal antibodies that recognize the surface of cariogenic bacteria. They used three highly species-specific monoclonal immunoglobulin G (IgG) antibodies targeted against *Streptococcus mutans*. The probes are tagged with fluorescent molecules that measure quantitatively with spectrometer.

Advantages include that it can be used at chairside by dentist, quick results, and the overall risk assessment can be made in operatory itself.

Shi *et al.* developed three highly species-specific monoclonal IgG antibodies against *S. mutans* that quantitatively detect *S. mutans* in <1 min and is sensitive enough to detect a single bacterial cell and concluded that these methods could be widely used in basic and clinical studies related to *S. mutans* and in the clinical diagnosis and treatment of caries in humans.

Gu *et al.* study showed that MAb-based salivary *S. mutans* tests exhibit significantly higher specificity and sensitivity than the commonly used selective culture method and thus provides useful information and tools for analyzing the role of *S. mutans* in human dental caries

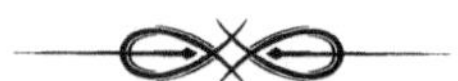

Caries Detecting Dyes

There are two layers of decalcification in carious dentin. The first one is the soft and infected layer which doesn't have the capacity of remineralization. The second one is hard, intermediately decalcified and has the ability of remineralization. Many studies were carried out to differentiate these layers. Although there are opinions stating the benefit of caries detection dyes, there are also opinions that dyes can lead to over-reduction in the dentin

Most clinical investigations have concluded that, caries detection dyes don't stain bacteria but stain the less mineralized organic matrix.

In a study of **Demarco** *et al.* they suggested that dye remnants that remained on the walls of the cavity may cause a decrease in the shear bond strength between the composite restorations and the enamel.

Y.Hosoya, T Taguchi , F R Tay in 2007 evaluated the clinical efficacy of a new caries detecting dye using a laser fluorescence device (DIAGNOdent).

Primary and permanent teeth with dentin caries were stained with Caries Check (CC), containing 1% acid red in polypropylene glycol (MW = 300) or Caries Detector (CD), containing 1% acid red in propylene glycol (MW= 76). Primary-CC, primary-CD, permanent-CC and permanent-CD groups were prepared. In the CC groups, stained dentin was completely removed. In the CD groups, pink-stained dentin was retained according to the manufacturers' instructions.[47] Cavities before and after caries removal were measured with the DIAGNOdent. Data were analyzed using ANOVA and Fisher's PLSD multiple comparison test at $\alpha = 0.05$.

The study concluded when dentin stained with Caries Check was completely removed, the DIAGNOdent readings were higher than those recorded when palely-stained pink dentin was retained with the Caries Detector, with significant difference observed for the permanent teeth.

Caries Check may be used clinically to avoid excessive removal of caries-affected or sound dentin in permanent teeth but not in primary teeth.

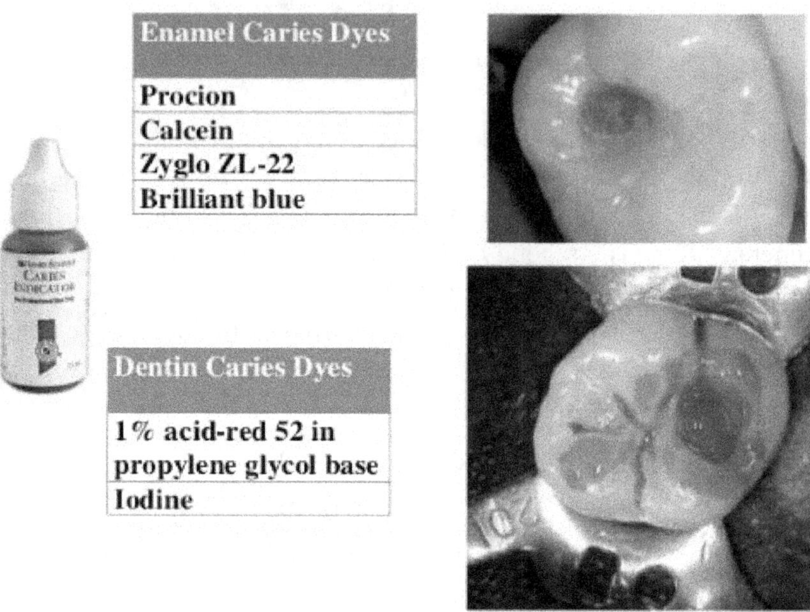

Figure 60: Caries Detector Dyes

Fluorescence Camera (VistaProof):

It is based on the light- induced fluorescence phenomenon. (Dürr Dental, Bietigheim-Bissingen, Germany) that is based on six blue GaN-LEDs emitting a 405-nm light. With this camera it is possible to digitize the video signal from the dental surface during fluorescence emission using a CCD sensor (charge coupled device).

On these images, it is possible to see different areas of the dental surface that fluoresce in green (sound dental tissue) and in red (carious dental tissue) . DBSWIN software is used to analyze the images and translate into values the intensity ratio of the red and green fluorescence. The software highlights the lesions and classifies them in a scale from 0 to 5, giving a treatment orientation in the first evaluation: monitoring, remineralization or invasive treatment.

Quantitative Light/Laser-Induced Fluorescence

The use of fluorescence for the detection of caries dates back to 1929 first described by Benedict. Fluorescence results from change in the characteristics of light caused by a change in wavelength of incident light rays following reflection from the surface of material.

QLF is based on the principle of fluorescence. It enhances early detection of carious lesions, particularly progression or regression of white spots of smooth surface lesions. It provides a fluorescent image of a tooth surface within yellow-green spectrum of visible light that quantifies mineral loss and size of the lesion .

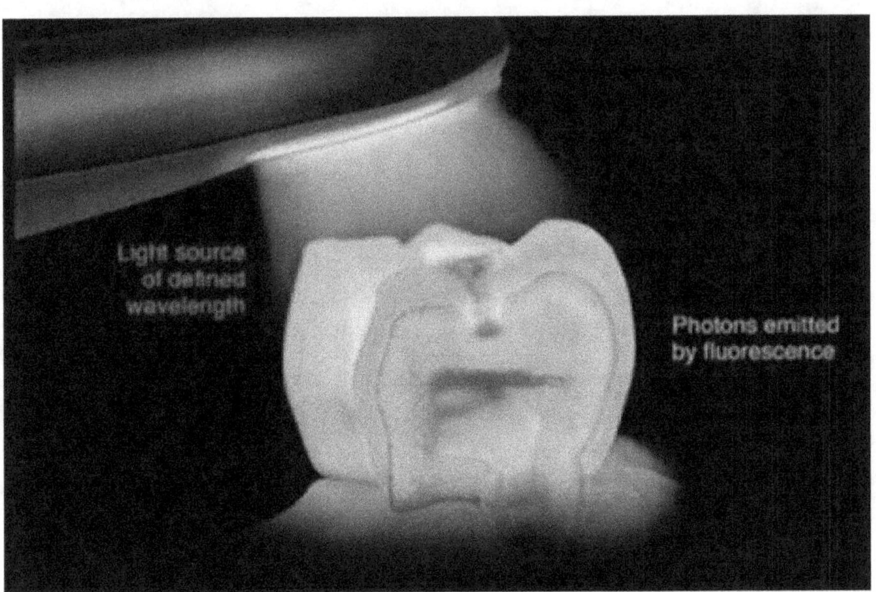

Figure 61: Quantitative Light/Laser-Induced Fluorescence

It is a suitable method for quantitative assessment of early enamel lesions in visually inaccessible areas. Most important parameters produced by QLF are lesion area, depth, and volume.

Ferreira Zandoná in 2010 conducted a study to combine a standardized visually based system, the International Caries Detection and Assessment System (ICDAS), with a sensitive fluorescence-based system, quantitative light-induced fluorescence (QLF) and to determine the ability to monitor caries lesion progression. This combination (QLF-I) has the potential to increase the sensitivity of the visual method without compromising specificity. A total of 460 children were enrolled and examined at baseline, 8 months and 12 months by ICDAS and QLF by a single examiner and DMFT score was 6.0 (SD 5.8) at baseline and 6.4 (SD 6.3) at 12 months, and both methods were able to follow the increase in incidence. The QLF-I scored more surfaces at the early ICDAS scores (1 and 2) and score 4. Not all lesions progressed at the same rate, differing by score at baseline and surface type.

Yin D.Y. Hu X. Fan assessed the ability of a new dentifrice containing arginine, an insoluble calcium compound, and fluoride to arrest or reverse naturally occurring buccal caries lesions measured using Quantitative Light-induced Fluorescence (QLF).[48] Three study groups used dentifrices which contained 1) 1.5% arginine and 1450 ppm fluoride as sodium monofluo- rophosphate (experimental), 2) 1450 ppm fluoride as sodium monofluorophosphate (positive control), and 3) no fluoride (negative control). All three dentifrices were formulated in the same calcium base. The study participants were from three schools in the city of Chengdu, Sichuan Province, China. A total of 446 of 450 recruited subjects completed the study. Of these, 147 were in the experi- mental, 148 in the positive control, and 151 in the negative control groups. The initial age of the children was 10–12 years (mean 11.4 ± 0.54); 47.5% were female. Using QLF, assessments of buccal caries lesions were made at baseline and after three and six months of product use. For DQ, representing lesion volume, the baseline mean value for the three groups was 27.30, and at the three-month examination the mean values were 16.76, 19.25, and 25.89 for the experimental, positive, and negative control dentifrices, respectively. This represents improvements from baseline of 38.6%, 29.5%, and 5.2%. At six months, the DQ values for the three groups were

13.46, 18.47, and 24.18, representing improvements from baseline of 50.7%, 32.3%, and 11.4%. For all QLF metrics, DF (loss of fluorescence), area,and DQ, the differences between the negative control and both the experimental and positive control groups were statistically significant(p ≤0.01).The differences between the experimental and positive control groups attained statistical significance for DQ

QLF uses the natural fluorescence of the teeth and depends on the light absorption and scattering properties of the teeth, to discriminate between caries and surrounding sound enamel. The auto-fluorescence of tooth tissue decreases with demineralization and QLF measures the percentage fluorescence change in demineralized enamel with respect to surrounding sound enamel and relates it to the amount of mineral lost during demineralization.[49]

Stookey reported that QLF can be used to assess the impact of preventive measures on the re-mineralization and reversal of the caries process as it is capable of monitoring and quantifying changes in the mineral content of white spot lesions.[50]

Ando *et al.* determined and compared the ability of QLF (laser) and QLF II (light) to quantify mineral loss from carious lesions in both deciduous and permanent teeth and concluded that the use of either QLF method to quantify mineral loss in early carious lesions in deciduous teeth is slightly more accurate in comparison to permanent teeth.[51]

Heinrich-Weltzien *et al.* concluded that QLF seems to be a sensitive method that is suitable for the detection of visually undetected initial caries lesions on all maxillary and mandibular smooth surfaces in caries-risk adolescents .[52]

Higham *et al.* concluded that "QLF has the potential to detect, diagnose, and longitudinally monitor occlusal caries and provides useful information to the clinician with regard to the severity of the lesion and likely treatment."

Unlu *et al.* compared LF device, electronic caries monitor (ECM), and caries detector dye and concluded that LF has significantly detected residual caries.[53]

Gimenez *et al.* performed a comprehensive systematic review and meta-analysis to evaluate the accuracy of fluorescence-based methods in detecting caries lesions. In general, the analysis demonstrated that the fluorescence- based method tends to have similar accuracy for detecting more advanced caries lesions on all types of teeth, dental surfaces, or settings.

Emineralization or remineralization.[54]

Mechanism Of Action

System includes a measurement probe, control unit, and computer fitted with a frame grabber. The control unit consists of an illumination device and imaging electronics. Light source is a special arc lamp based on xenon technology. The light from this lamp is filtered by a blue-transmitting filter.

A liquid light guide transports blue light to the teeth. Recording of florescent image is done with a yellow transmitting filter positioned in front of the color CCD sensor. Image is then digitized by the frame grabber and is available for quantitative analysis. Tooth is seen on a computer monitor as fluorescent green and dark areas indicate mineral loss or white spot lesions. Image can be saved and compared over time to track d .

This technique is based on the principle that as the mineral content of the tooth changes the auto fluorescence of the tooth changes also. The light scatters much faster in carious tissues compared to sound dental tissues, shortening the pathway of the light in the lesion and decreasing the absorption and fluorescence in this area. This means that, the scattering of the light is used for evaluating the mineral loss related with the lesion . It can also be used in measuring the red fluorescence from microorganisms in plaque. The value of red fluorescence can be used in the evaluation of oral hygiene, assessment of the plaque on the dentures, detection of the infected dentin and detecting the leakage of a sealant or caries at the margin of a restoration .

The QLF method was suggested as an efficient technique not only for the detection early caries but also monitoring the progression of a lesion or remineralization process .

QLF uses the natural fluorescence of the teeth and depends on the light absorption and scattering properties of the teeth, to discriminate between caries and surrounding sound enamel. The auto-fluorescence of tooth tissue decreases with demineralization and QLF measures the percentage fluorescence change in demineralized enamel with respect to surrounding sound enamel and relates it to the amount of mineral lost during demineralization.

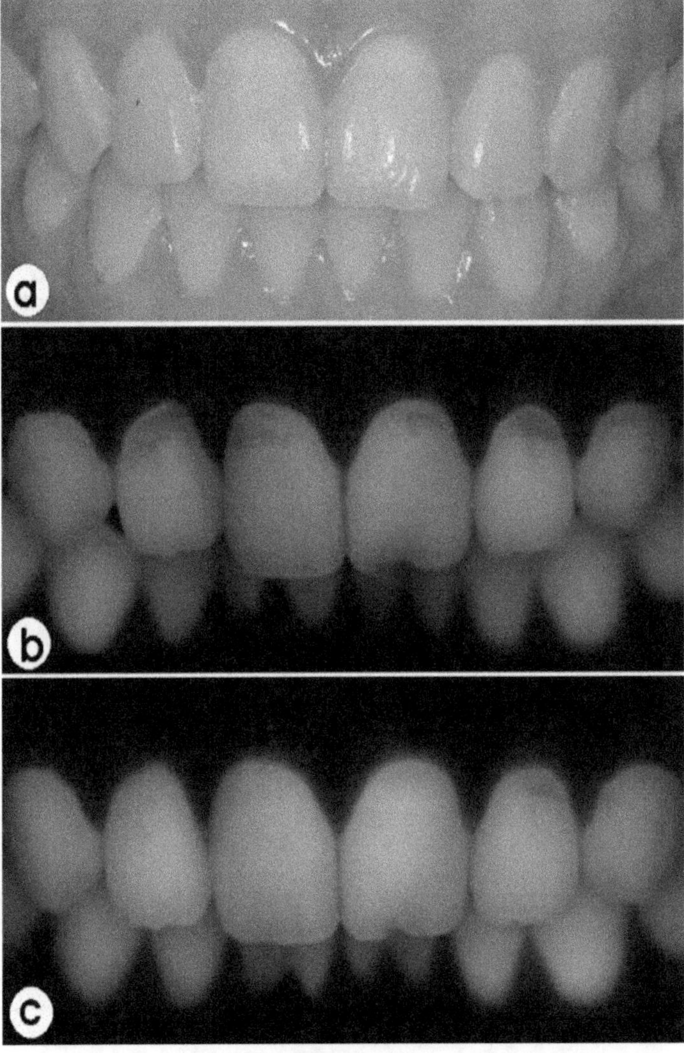

Figure 62: QLF

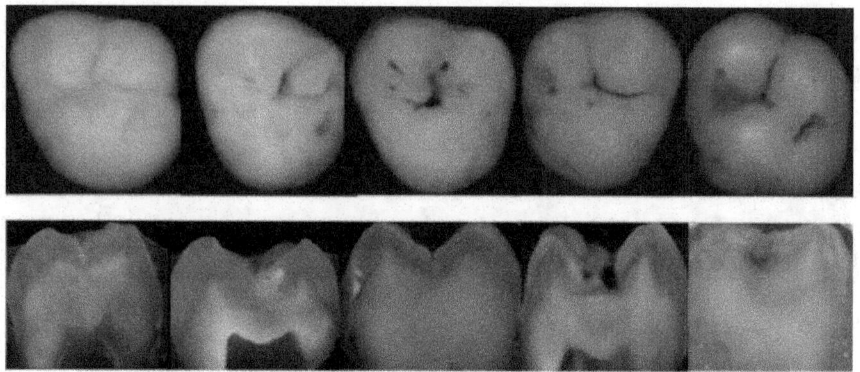

Figure 63: QLF Images Compared With Histological Sections

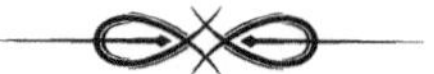

Ultrasonics (Ultrasound Caries Detector)

Use of ultrasound to detect dental caries has been proposed for the past 30 years, but the technique has received renewed interest particularly in the past 10 years. It was introduced for detecting early carious lesions on smooth surfaces.

Demineralization of natural enamel is assessed by ultrasound pulse-echo technique. It is observed that there is a definite correlation between the mineral content of the body of the lesion and the relative echo amplitude changes.

Principle

Ultrasound makes the use of sound waves with frequency. They are longitudinal or pressure waves which travel through gasses, liquids, and solids. Ultrasound interacts differently with different tissues.

They have a frequency of $>20,000$ Hz and have all the properties of waves, in that they may be reflected, scattered, refracted, or absorbed. The relative ability of a medium to reflect sound depends on its mechanical properties such as elasticity, density, and wavelength of sound.

Amount of sound reflected provides information about the structure of reflecting interface, whereas the time taken for sound to be reflected provides information about the position of the reflecting interface. Sound waves produced as a result of minute changes in crystal dimension may be omitted continually, as burst of waves or as a single pulse.

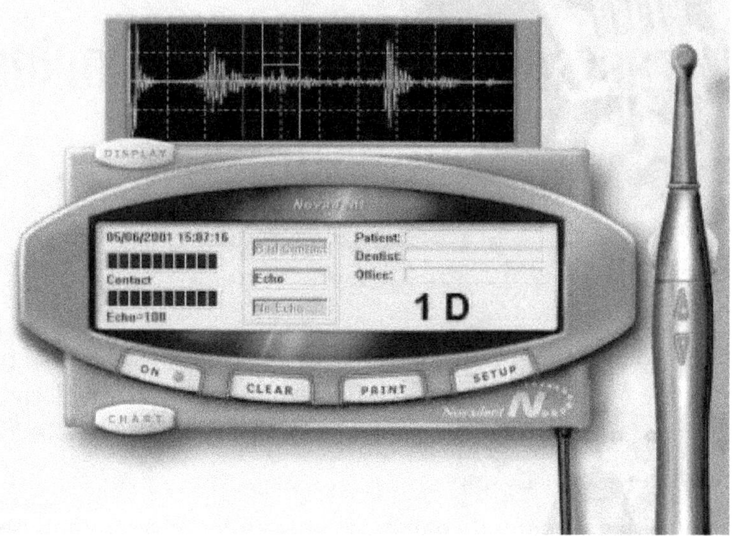

Figure 64: Ultrasound Detector

Mechanism Of Action

For sound waves to reach the tooth, they have to travel through a coupling medium or an agent which has acoustic impedance. Various acoustic coupling agents have been used such as mercury, aluminum rods, water, and glycerin.

An ultrasonic probe is used which sends and receives longitudinal waves to and from the surface of the tooth. Initial white spot lesions produce no or weak surface echoes, whereas sites with visible cavitation produce echoes with substantially higher amplitude.

This method if improved can be a realistic alternative to radiographic diagnosis of caries on approximal surfaces. It is also more sensitive than visual-tactile method.

Sound waves can be used for the detection of caries. Ultrasound can detect lesions easily because the travel time of ultrasonic pulses differ in sound and demineralized enamel tissues . This method is considered promising in detecting early enamel lesions because the white spot lesions confined to enamel produce no detectable or weak echoes whereas deeper lesions produce substantially higher amplitudes .

Thermography

A liquid crystal thermography uses a thermometer consisting of flexible rubber sheets and cholesteric crystal which are arranged in several layers and are mounted in a frame. These sheets also have the provision for inflation so that the heat-sensitive surface conforms better to the body's contour. To measure the thermal changes, the crystal sheets are placed over the surfaces to be examined. After placement, the crystals change from their neutral color into different color in response to the surface temperature. The resultant color display is then photographed using polaroid photography which gives an instant hard copy of the image.

IR was first discovered by Sir William Herschel in 1800 and it was his son Sir John F. W. Herschel who recorded these spectra on the infra side of red around 1840. All objects including the human body emit radiation in the infrared spectrum, and according to Wien's law, the frequency at which the maximum energy is emitted is dependent on the temperature of the body

This method allows the examination of dark areas in the bottom of the pits and fissures. If a darkened area is considered as decay, the abrasion technology is used to deliver alumina particles to the suspicious area. If this darkened area is stain or organic plug, it will be cleaned by abrasion leaving the sound tissue behind .

Usually after the bursting of the particles the underlying decay masked by the stain is revealed. This undetected caries may even be a deep lesion. Further application of abrasion can be used to remove the caries until the healthy tooth structure is revealed

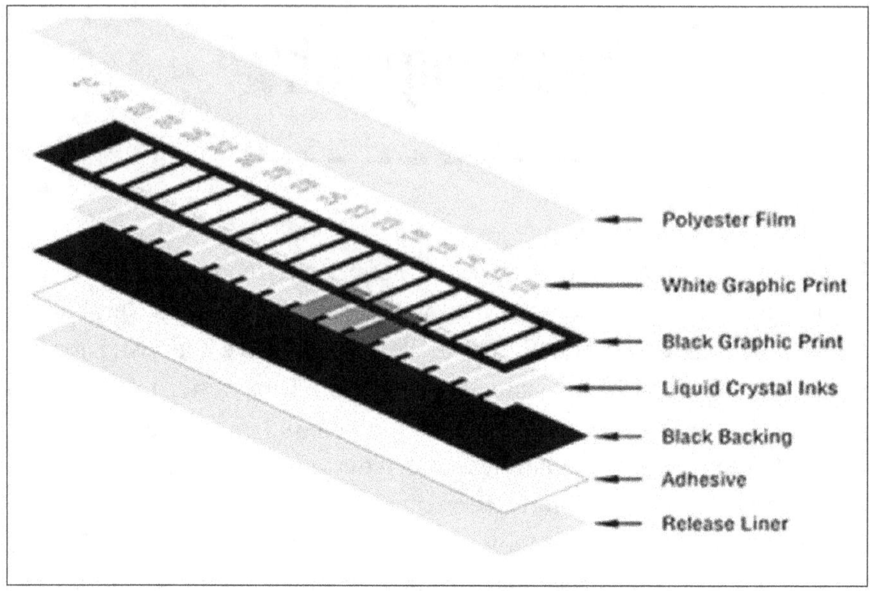

Figure 65: Crystal thermography

Terahertz Imaging

This method uses waves in terahertz frequency (1012 Hz or a wavelength of 30 μm). This wavelength is short enough to provide reasonable resolution but long enough to prevent loss of signal due to scattering . Several advantages of this system are as follows ;

Human tissue is relatively transparent to terahertz rays,

- Low powers are used for imaging,

- Non-ionizing radiation is used,

- The electrical charge of the tissues examined remain unchanged,

- The images are clear but due to long wavelength of the source spatial resolution is low.

Studies concerning this method of imaging are limited but promising.

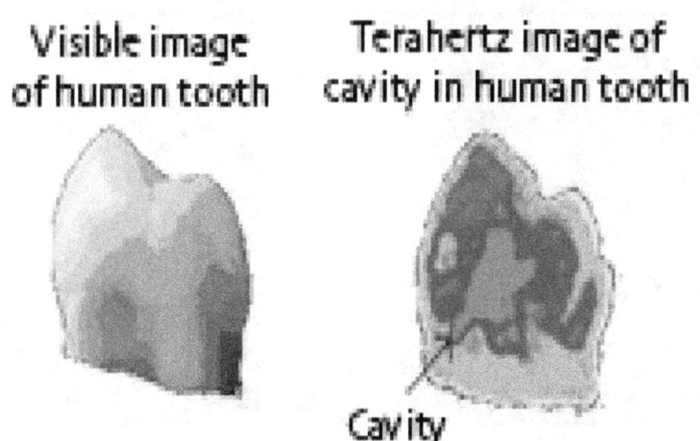

Figure 66: Tetrahertz Imaging

Multiphoton Imaging

Infrared light of 850 nm wavelength is used in this imaging technique. While conventional fluorescence imaging uses a single blue photon to excite fluorescence compound of the tooth, multi photon imaging uses two infrared photons (with half the energy of the blue photon) which are absorbed simultaneously. With this technique, sound tooth structure shows strong fluorescence whereas carious tissues fluoresce weaker. The carious regions appear as dark areas in strongly fluorescing tooth.

Infrared Fluorescence

There are limited studies regarding this technique. In theory, the tooth is irradiated with 700-15000 nm wavelength light. Barrier filters are used to measure the resulting fluorescence.

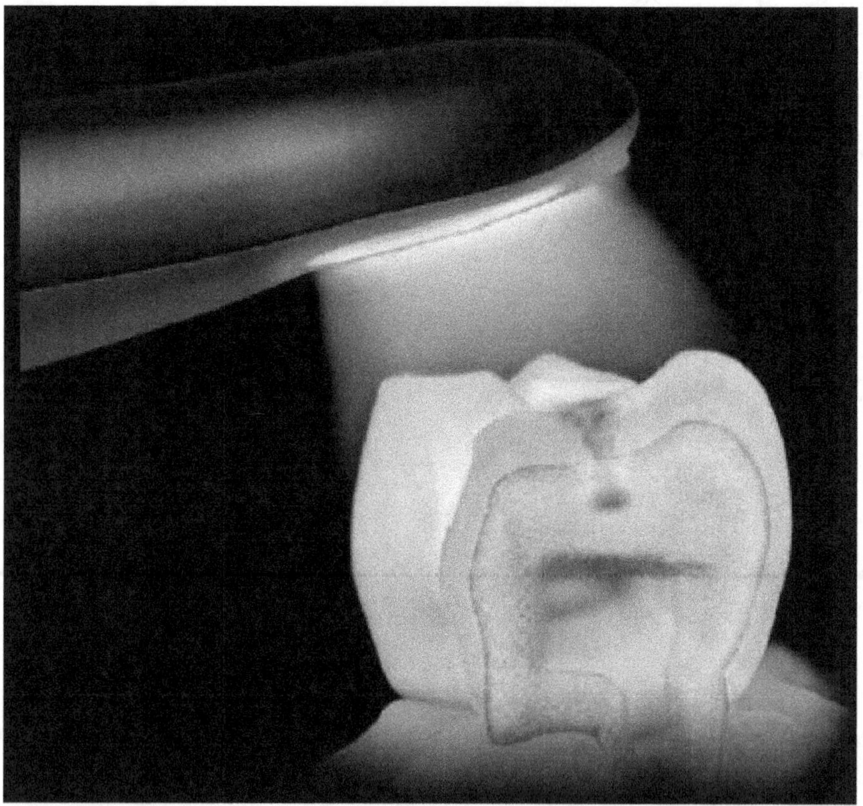

Figure 67: Flourescence

Led Technology For Caries Diagnosis

The technology is based on the principle of fluorescence, where a specific wavelength of light shines on the tooth and is then reflected back in 2 basic colors: green when the dentin is healthy, and red when the dentin is infected. A device that combines high magnification intraoral imaging with fluorescence becomes a powerful time-saving tool for diagnosing and proposing treatment. The same device can then guide the clinician through the treatment of caries removal. This process has been named light-induced fluorescence evaluation for diagnosis and treatment (LIFEDT).

The **SOPROLIFE Camera** (ACTEON North America) is a new intraoral LED camera working as 2 devices in one; operating as an intraoral camera as well as a caries detection device. Patients who are routinely seen in hygiene and exam areas with the question in their mind, "Will my dentist find something today?" will find the diagnosis of early caries of asymptomatic teeth much easier to process. A moment of truth or trust issue at the time of this diagnosis can be much easier with this unique intraoral camera showing the patient through magnification the carious grooves and suspicious shadows of interproximal decay. An explanation of the fluorescence concept and reference colors facilitates a co-diagnostic experience.

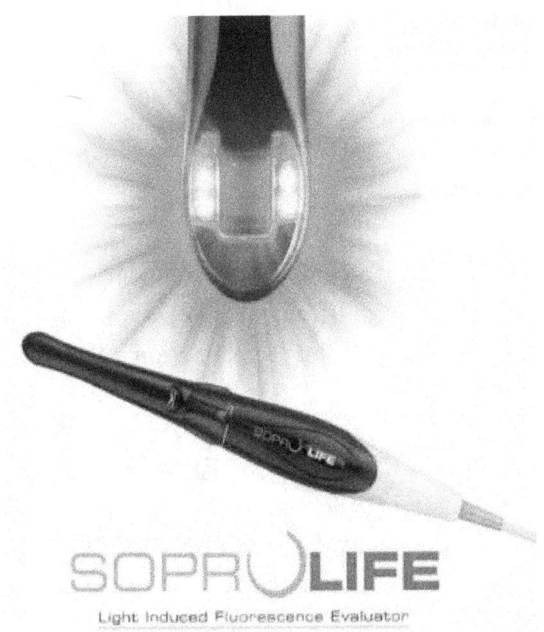

Figure 68: Soprolife

For the dentist, use of the fluorescence mode becomes a treatment aid to differentiate diseased versus healthy tissue. Another benefit to using the

SOPROLIFE camera is that a history of carious lesions can be documented, and changes in their development can guide treatment decisions. Instead of informing patients that you will "watch" this tooth, a pictorial reference is easily made into the patient record.

Science Of Fluorescence And Autofluorescence

Fluorescence is the emission of light by a substance that has absorbed light or other electromagnetic radiation of a different wavelength. Dental tissues have fluorescent molecules (fluorophores or fluorchromes) which absorb light, then emit the energy back as fluorescent light—this is called autofluorescence. This process was described by Banerjee, et al5 in 2000. It became the basis for a new method of diagnosing initial caries. Scientists and clinical researchers at SOPRO, a company specializing in dental imaging, found that a blue LED emitting light at 450 nm was able optimize the autofluorescence of the dental structures. The fluorescence signal reflected was extremely low intensity compared to the 450 nm intensity sent by the blue LEDs. By amplifying the fluorescent signal, a new level of tissue distinction could be made.

Healthy dentin could be clearly discriminated from carious dentin as it fluoresced a bright green signal. The wavelength of the autofluorescence signal varies according to the density and chemical composition of the surface tissue and subsurface. The determination was made that that one of either the inorganic or organic constituents of healthy dentin that emits the acid-green fluorescence partially disappeared during the caries process; subsequently, a red fluorescence signal would appear. The autofluorescence technology allowed detection of early occlusal, even interproximal, decay.

LED Camera Operation And Suggested Use

The camera has a magnification range of more than 50x. Using this magnification reveals anatomy far more precisely then visual and hand probing.6 The use of conventional probing has also been considered controversial based on the possibility of "inoculating" or transferring lesion contents.

The camera has 3 modes: the daylight mode, the diagnostic mode, and the treatment mode. The daylight mode has 4 settings which allow clear images for portraits, smiles, intraoral and macro views.

The diagnostic mode, labeled mode I on the images, filters out colors of the surrounding soft tissues of the mouth, rendering them black and white. It amplifies and displays in color the fluorescence signal response sent by the dentin. A healthy tooth appears white with a homogeneous green hue on top of it. The diagnostic mode is focused more on enamel. Differences in thickness of enamel as well as material deposits will affect the fluorescence response. Thicker enamel reduces the fluorescence response and gives a slightly blue image. Demineralized enamel gives a white, color-free response. Since demineralization is the first stage of the caries destruction, noting white colors can be very important.7

Significant amount of material deposits tend to give a black signal, which is considered an alert to clean the deposits and reassess the signal. Infected dentin gives a dark red autofluorescence signal. Incipient and evolving lesions magnified in the diagnostic mode tend to have mixed signal colors of red centers surrounded by black grooves and green islands. This is because material deposits shown as black can minimize the red signal of dentin caries.

The treatment mode, labeled mode II on the images, also filters out the surrounding soft tissues of the mouth, rendering them black and white. This mode also amplifies and displays in color the fluorescence signal of the dentin. The only difference in the treatment mode is that the red wavelengths are amplified more and the blue wavelengths are decreased. Carious dentin gives a red fluorescence signal so the amplified red color in the treatment modes assists in the excavation process—a photographic caries detector of sorts.

Tables 1 and 2 summarize the signal colors and their relevance to tissue characteristics.

Methods And Materials

Clinicians continue to be confronted with how to identify carious tissue and when to stop the caries excavation process. The goal of these case studies was to evaluate a protocol using LIFEDT with the SOPROLIFE

Camera for caries treatment decisions as to when to treat and to what extent the caries removal should be performed. In addition, we compared use of the SOPROLIFE camera in the treatment mode to the use of caries dye indicators with the assumption light evaluation could expedite the excavation process by eliminating the repetitive cycle of dye application and rinsing.

The Protocol:

1. Initial observation of suspicious grooves, fissures, and shadows in the daylight, then diagnostic modes.

2. Fluorescence analysis and therapeutic decision with the diagnostic mode.

3. Radiographic evaluation/correlation.

4. Fluorescence assisted lesion removal in treatment mode.

5. Restorative treatment.

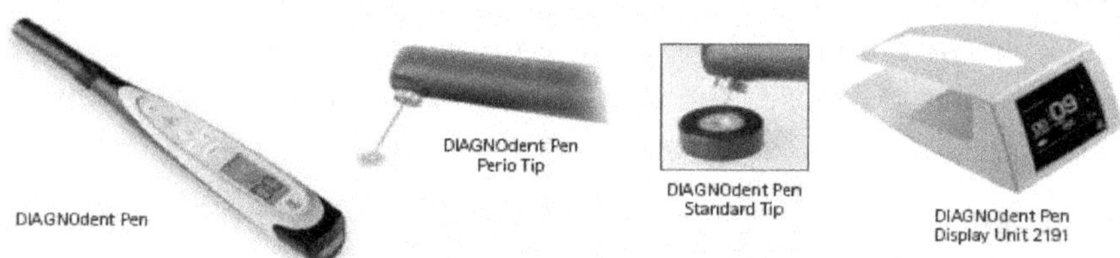

Figure 69: Diagnodent

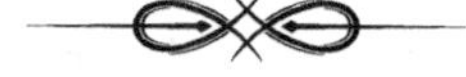

Salivary Protein Biomarkers Of Caries Risk

The first attempts to relate the protein composition of human saliva and the risk of caries were based on the determination of the total protein concentration. Generally, the total protein content in saliva was increased with caries activity; however, no differences attributable to caries activity were confirmed in several experimental studies published to date. The total protein concentration variable failed as a simple test of caries susceptibility. [55] It has become clear that more than the total concentration of proteins, the qualitative composition of salivary proteins plays an important role. A number of studies have also been carried out to investigate the protein profile of the saliva of healthy individuals compared to salivary samples of patients with dental caries using electrophoretic analysis. In one study , the authors qualitatively analyzed protein profiles of whole unstimulated human saliva by SDS-PAGE attempting to find a correlation with the decayed, missing, and filled teeth index (DMFT). The identification of proteins according to the criteria described by revealed no significant dissimilarities between men and women, and only minimal correlation between the total protein concentrations in both genders. Regarding the salivary proteins of individuals with a high-level DMFT status, substantial down-regulation or the absence of mucin-1, mucin-2, and the acidic PRP-1 were found. The composition of proteins in whole human saliva of subjects with the active dental caries was also studied by Roa *et al.* by comparing the individuals with filled caries cavities and the CF subjects. Electrophoretic assessment showed that the composition of proteins is very similar in all groups with the exception of 17 kDa protein, present in males with active dental caries. In another study , the etiology of early childhood caries (ECC) was examined. SDS-PAGE gels manifested a considerable degree of resemblance between the proteomes of children's saliva with ECC and a control CF group, which was in contrast with expectations. On the other hand, in the study of caries in early childhood individuals the increased number of bands of PRPs was determined by SDS-PAGE and correlated significantly with entities without tooth decay, which according to the authors, is linked with the protective effect of PRPs.

Immunoglobulins

In the last decade, a number of candidate proteins that have the potential to be diagnostic and prognostic biomarkers for dental caries have been examined. A great deal of attention is being paid to the various immunoglobulins that constitute the major group of proteins of human saliva.[56] The prominent immunoglobulins in saliva are a subclass of immunoglobulin A (IgA) or the dimeric form of IgA, also called secretory IgA (s-IgA), followed by immunoglobulin G (IgG) and immunoglobulin M (IgM) subclasses. S-IgA is abundant in the mucosal secretions. Salivary s-IgA is postulated to be a factor that protects against dental caries by controlling the growth of cariogenic oral microflora, preventing pathogen adhesion and the activation of bacterial enzymes and toxins. S-IgA is a primary molecule responding to a stimulus in the salivary environment, i.e., s-IgA is a protein responsible for adaptive immunity. According to such IgA-mediated immunity can be induced most efficiently via the mucosal route rather than by any systemic method.

s-IgA action:

According to one theory, the s-IgA in the saliva of caries-susceptible patients is reduced due to the binding to cariogenic microbiota, whereas according to another model, binding leads to the secretory immune response, resulting in an increase in free s-IgA.

Numerous investigations have reported contradictory results with respect to the correlation of salivary s-IgA with dental caries. The analysis of s-IgA content in saliva using enzyme immunoassay established that in healthy patients, average values were significantly higher than in patients with caries of contact surfaces of lateral teeth, implying an effective defense function of s-IgA . Similarly, s-IgA tends to be higher in CF status, with no statistically significant differences between rheumatoid arthritis and nonrheumatoid arthritis individuals.

On the other hand, an investigation by **Liu *et al.*** demonstrated the positive correlation of the chemokine CCL28 and s-IgA content in saliva with dental caries in children. According to the authors, children's dental decay leads to the secretion of chemokine CCL28, which promotes the secretion of s-IgA. Likewise, whole s-IgA levels of children were significantly higher in the group with DMFT≥3 compared with the group with DMFT=0. Parissoto *et al.* showed that the secretory immune system of children at 3-4 years is undergoing significant maturation. At baseline, the salivary IgA concentration of the caries group was higher than that of the CF group. Over the study period, an increase in salivary IgA in both groups was observed, although IgA concentration only changed significantly in the CF group. Simultaneously, a significant increase in salivary IgA antibody levels to glucosyltransferase, glucan-binding protein (Gbp) and antigen I/II salivary binding region was detected. Controversially, children with s-ECC simultaneously with high *S. mutans* colonization presented a decrease in salivary IgA impact on *S. mutans* GbpB, demonstrating the possible effect of this immunologically dominant protein on the extent of tooth decay in childhood .Some authors, on the other hand, observed no change in s-IgA levels related to the caries index of children with diabetes mellitus .Thus, the available evidence demonstrates conflicting and inconclusive results regarding the IgA content in CA samples and CF controls.

Frequency domain infrared photothermal radiometry and modulated luminescence

Although still under development, the most recent technology in the field of caries diagnosis is the combined frequency-domain laser-induced infrared photothermal radiometry and modulated luminescence PTR/LUM. Some of the inherent advantages of the adaptation of PTR to dental diagnosis in conjunction with LUM emission as the dualprobe technique have been reported in recent literature. The PTR technique is based on the modulated thermal infrared blackbody or Planck radiation response of a medium, resulting from optical radiation absorption from a lowintensity laser beam and optical-to-thermal energy conversion followed by modulated temperature rise "thermal waves" usually less than 1 °C in magnitude. The generated signals from PTR/LUM instrument carry subsurface information in the form of a spatially damped temperature. Thus PTR has depth-profilometric ability i.e it can penetrate and yield information about an opaque or highly scattering medium well beyond the range of optical imaging. The laser-intensity modulation-frequency dependence of the penetration depth of thermal waves makes it possible to perform depth profiling of materials.

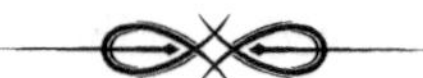

Canary System

A Canary Number is the output generated by The Canary System to inform the oral health care professional about the probable health status of a given tooth. Using a complex algorithm, The Canary System converts the unique PTR/LUM signatures into a Canary Number on a scale from 0 to 100 which appears on a monitor screen and is also audible. Lower numbers suggest healthy enamel and higher numbers suggest the presence of cracks and caries.

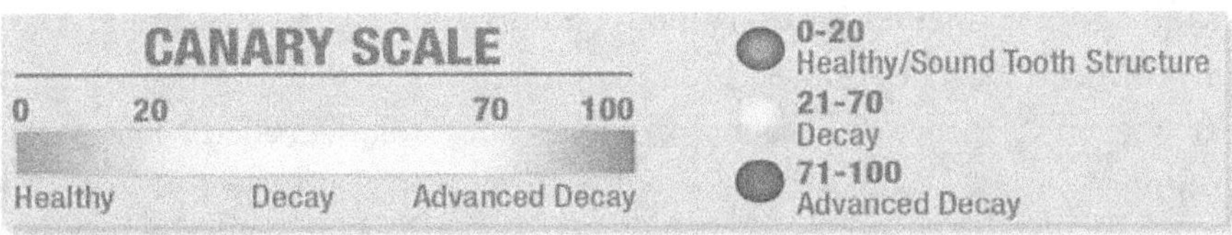

Figure 70: Canary Scale

For proximal caries diagnosis, The Canary System is more accurate than bitewing radiography. The Canary had a sensitivity of 92% compared to 67% for bitewing radiography, according to an independent human clinical study conducted at the University of Texas and released at the International Association for Dental Research Meeting in March 2015.

The Canary System can detect cracks and caries that are not seen with other devices and do require treatment. Patients become engaged in their treatment and understand the need for operative intervention.

Canary System is the only caries detection system that:

- Analyzes and measures the crystal structure of the tooth

- Measures up to a depth of 5 mm

- Detects decay on all tooth surfaces including:

  - ➤ Around and beneath the intact margins of restorations including amalgam, composites and crowns

- Smooth surfaces,

- Occlusal pits and fissures, including beneath stained areas

- Around orthodontic brackets

- Interproximal regions

- Beneath opaque and transparent dental sealants

The Canary System is bridged to most practice management software. Abrams SH, Sivagurunathan KS, Silvertown JD et al correlated lesion depth of natural caries, measured with Polarized Light Microscopy (PLM), to Canary Numbers (CN) derived from The Canary System™ (CS), numerical readings from DIAGNOdent (DD), and lesion scores from ICDAS II.A total of 20 examination sites on extracted human molars and premolars were selected. The selected examination sites consisted of healthy and enamel caries on smooth and occlusal surfaces of each tooth. Two blinded dentists ranked each examination site using ICDAS II and the consensus score for each examined site was recorded. The same examination sites were scanned with CS and DD, and the CN and DD readings were recorded. After all the measurements were completed, the readings of the three caries detection methods were validated with a histological method, Polarized Light Microscopy (PLM). PLM performed by blinded examiners was used as the 'gold standard' to confirm the presence or absence of a caries lesion within each examined site and to determine caries lesion depth.[57]

A study demonstrated that the CS exhibits much higher correlation with caries lesion depth compared to ICDAS II and DD. CS may provide the clinician with more information about the size and position of the lesion which might help in monitoring or treating the lesion.The present extracted tooth study found that The Canary System correlates with caries lesion depth more accurately that ICDAS II and DIAGNOdent.

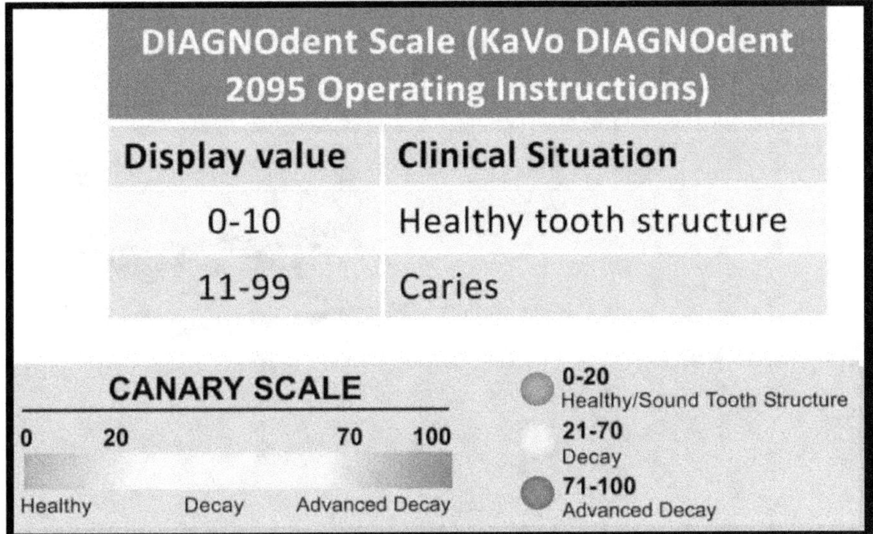

Figure 71: DIAGNOdent Scale And Canary Scale

Canary System is a precise, low-powered, laser-based instrument with an integrated intraoral camera that detects the presence of cracks and caries (tooth decay) before they are large enough to appear on dental X-rays. Intraoral camera images can be displayed for immediate chair side review with the patient. A patient report is generated containing an odontogram with Canary Numbers, which are color-coded for the examined teeth, along with the dentist's treatment recommendation.

Principle :

When placed on the tooth surface, a low-powered, pulsating laser light is shone on the tooth during a 3 second scan. The pulses of laser light generate photothermal (PTR) and luminescence (LUM) responses. By using a laser pulse at a frequency of 2Hz, the laser light can penetrate below the tooth surface and permit detection of a carious lesion as small as 50 microns (20 times smaller than a millimeter) and as deep as 5 mm from the tooth surface.

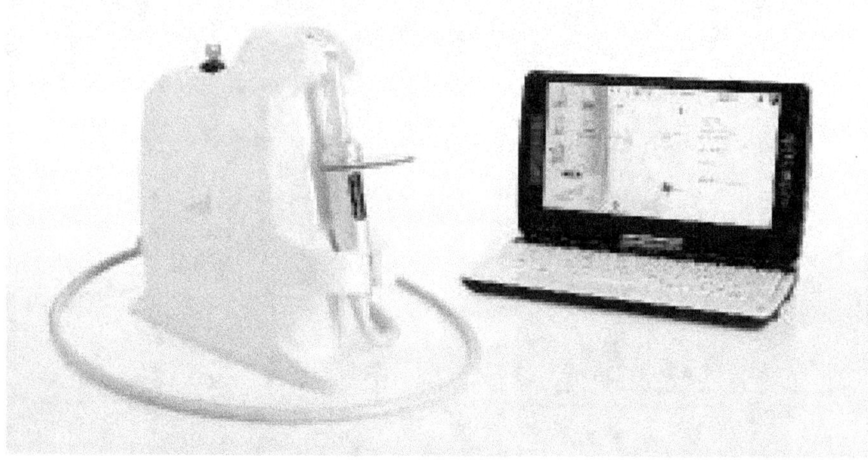

Figure 72: PTR

Traditional diagnostic technologies, visual inspection, manual probing and X-rays, are of little use if the decayed area is very small or below the tooth surface. They limit the ability of dentists to detect and monitor the early stages of tooth decay.

- **X-Rays**
  - ➤ The Canary System does not use ionizing radiation.

  - ➤ X-rays can only find caries on proximal surfaces once the lesion has grown to involve ½ the thickness of enamel. Radiographs can't detect lesions on smooth or occlusal surfaces until the lesions is very large

  - ➤ For proximal caries detection, The Canary System is more accurate than bitewing radiography.

- **Visual Inspection:**
  - ➤ Caries starts as a small lesion beneath the enamel surface. Visual inspection only examines the tooth surface and may find white or brown spots but visually one can't determine what has caused these surface changes.

- **Explorers and Manual Probing:**

  - Manual probing can damage tooth structure including pits and fissures and introduce bacteria deep into the pits and fissures of the teeth

Selecting The Right Caries Detection System:

Detecting and treating caries is one of the major therapeutic interventions of clinical practice. Selecting the right caries detection system can be very challenging and wrong choices can lead to wrong treatment decisions. The marketplace is filled with "claims" and information but how do you make sense of it all? We recommend that you ensure that the technology is actually detecting caries and other defects in the tooth structure.

Most technologies on the market today use fluorescence, which permits the detection of some surface bacteria. Fluorescence-based devices cannot give you any information about the crystal structure of the tooth. Fluorescence does not give any information about lesion size or depth. Fluorescence can only penetrate 0.5 mm beneath the tooth surface due to scattering of light from stain, plaque, organic deposits and surface features such as pits and fissures.

Fluorescence is simply the glow from an object that has absorbed light, such as light from LEDs or from specific wavelengths of lasers.

The literature indicates that bacterial by-products or porphyrins, stain, tartar and food debris all fluoresce under the wavelengths used in these devices, whether or not caries is present. Stained fissures that are healthy will fluoresce. Some toothpastes, polishing pastes, sealants and restorative materials have been shown to produce fluorescence, all resulting in false-positive readings.

Another technology on the market is transillumination which involves shining white and near-infrared light on a tooth to detect voids in the tooth. Two key limitations with this technique are: 1) No quantitative measurement is produced; and 2) Subjective interpretation of whether a dark area on the gray-scale images is caries or a dental anomaly leads to many false positives.

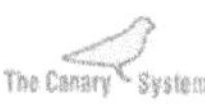

Cavity Detection Systems
- Clinical Comparison -

PRODUCT	Canary System	DIAGNOdent	Spectra	SoproLife	CariVu
MANUFACTURER	The Canary System by Quantum Dental Technologies	KaVo	AIR TECHNIQUES	ACTEON	DEXIS CariVu
Detects caries and cracks on all tooth surfaces	✓	✗	✗	✗	Interproximal Only
Detects caries under sealants – clear & opaque	✓	✗	✗	✗	✗
Detects sub-surface caries	✓	✗	✗	✗	✗
Detects & measures tooth structure beneath White/Brown spots	✓	✗	✗	✗	✗
Detects caries around margins of restorations (amalgam, composite, crowns & Glass Ionomer)	✓	Not accurate Measures porphyrins	Restorative materials glow preventing view of margin	Restorative materials glow preventing view of margin	Only large interproximal lesion at gingival margin
Detects caries around orthodontic brackets	✓	✗	✗	✗	✗
Quantifies changes in lesion size & volume	✓	Not accurate Measures porphyrins	Not accurate Measures porphyrins Small scale	Image Only no measurements	Subjective Observation of black/white image
Monitors & creates reports on the effectiveness of remineralization agents	✓	✗	✗	✗	✗

Table 18: Difference Between Canary System, Diagnodent, Spectra, Soprolife, Carivu

The Canary System is an evidence-based caries detection system built upon a solid foundation of peer-reviewed lab and clinical research. To review the research click here.

The Canary System allows dentists to identify decay that would have otherwise gone undetected. A small restoration can avoid the costly and uncomfortable procedures associated with large caries. With early detection, decay can be treated with remineralization therapies and potentially reversed. Restorations do not last a lifetime, and there is a cycle of continued placement and replacement of fillings. Caries can also develop under sealants. The Canary System can detect decay around and beneath the margins of fillings and under sealants.

Aids :
- It aids in detection of cracks and decay without exposure to ionizing radiation from Xrays and is comfortable and safe for young children.

- Provides early detection of small caries (cavities)that can be remineralized avoiding the placement of a filling

- Early detection and treatment of small caries and decay under old restorations or sealants and prevents their deep progression.

The **Canary Cloud** is an online, secure environment that allows Canary dentists to:

- View Canary scan data for each patient by tooth number and surface over a given time period and quickly generate customized reports

- Generate graphs of Canary Numbers over time for patients by tooth surface.

- Track Canary Scan usage in the office

- Keep up-to-date on Canary products, research, clinical news and order supplies

- Provide access to online training videos, manuals and presentations.

- Provides patient access to their own Canary reports with their own unique password.

The "canary in the mineshaft" was used for centuries to protect people from undetectable **hazards**. Today, the word is synonymous with an early warning system or alert. Patients will recognize The Canary System™ as a painless, less expensive, friendly (hand-held tool, ergonomic ease and function, yellow in colour) detection system for cavities that reduces the need for painful fillings and needles.

The Canary System™ is now available in the USA and Canada.

Abrams SH, Sivagurunathan *et al* correlated lesion depth of natural caries, measured with Polarized Light Microscopy (PLM), to Canary Numbers (CN) derived from The Canary System™ (CS), numerical readings from DIAGNOdent (DD), and lesion scores from ICDAS II. A total of 20 examination sites on extracted human molars and premolars were selected. The selected examination sites consisted of healthy and enamel caries on smooth and occlusal surfaces of each tooth. Two blinded dentists ranked each examination site using ICDAS II and the consensus score for each examined site was recorded. The same examination sites were scanned with CS and DD, and the CN and DD readings were recorded. After all the measurements were completed, the readings of the three caries detection methods were validated with a histological method, Polarized Light Microscopy (PLM). PLM performed by blinded examiners was used as the 'gold standard' to confirm the presence or absence of a caries lesion within each examined site and to determine caries lesion depth.The present extracted tooth study found that The Canary System correlates with caries lesion depth more accurately that ICDAS II and DIAGNOdent.[58]

The Canary System uses energy conversion technology (PTR-LUM) to image and examine the tooth. Pulses of laser light are aimed at the tooth, and the light is then converted to heat (Photothermal Radiometry or PTR) and light (luminescence or LUM), which are emitted from the tooth surface in response to the modulated pulses. These pulses of laser light enable the clinician to examine lesions up to 5 mm below the surface . Caries modifies the thermal properties (PTR) and luminescence (LUM) of healthy teeth. As a lesion grows, there is a corresponding change in the PTR LUM response signal. In effect, the heat confined to the region with crystalline disintegration (dental caries) increases the PTR and decreases the LUM response signal. As remineralization progresses and enamel prisms start to reform their structure, the thermal and luminescence properties begin to revert towards those of healthy tooth structure.

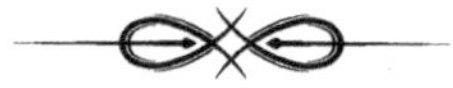

Face (Fluorescence-Aided Caries Excavation)

Blumer S, Kharouba J, compared the effectiveness of visual examination, radiographic examination and fluorescence-aided caries excavation (FACE) in detecting occlusal caries in first permanent molars in 150 children aged 6-14 years with intact occlusal surface with caries lesions without cavitation, or with darkened or deep fissures that had no clear diagnosis.

Two dentists independently performed a visual oral examination, FACE and bitewing radiography. The inter-rater reliability of each detection method was determined and their specificity and sensitivity.

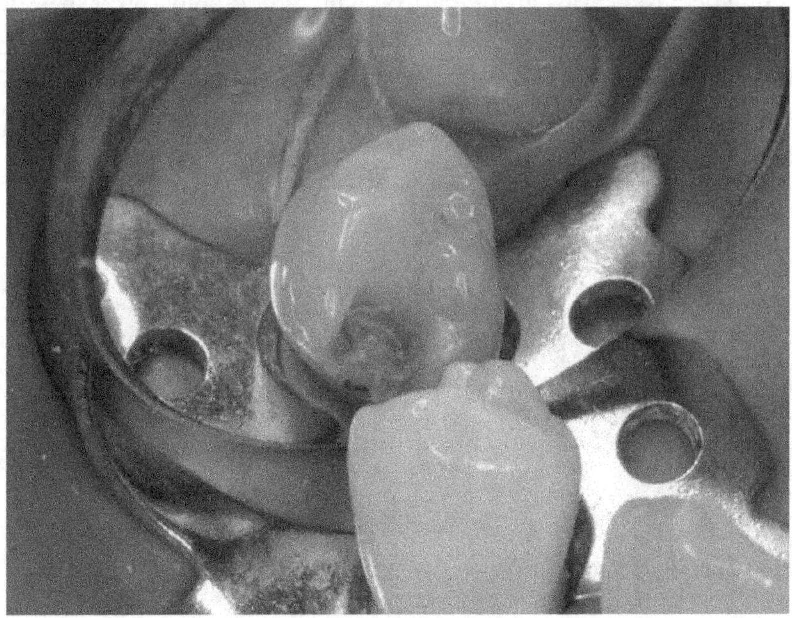

Figure 73: FACE For Detecting Caries

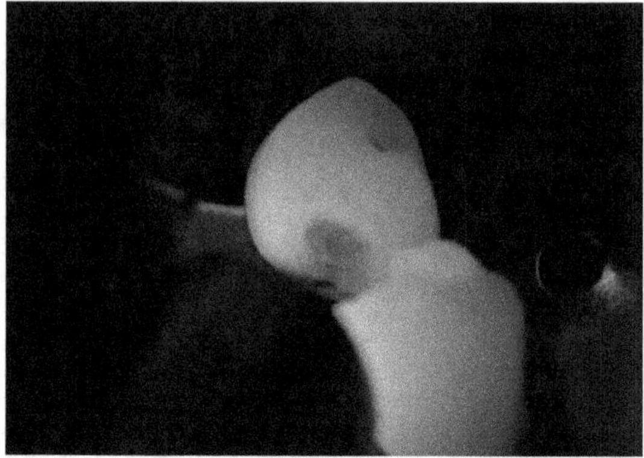

Figure 74: FACE detecting caries

All caries detection methods showed high inter-rater reliability with absolute agreement between raters above 90%. Most caries lesions were detected by visual (75.8%) and FACE (79.1%), while only 28.8% of lesions were detected by radiography. Detection by visual examination was strongly correlated with detection by FACE. A lower, yet statistically significant, correlation was found between visual examination and X-ray radiography .FACE had higher sensitivity (87%) and specificity (65%) for detecting occlusal caries in comparison with radiography (60% specificity and 55% sensitivity).The study concluded visual examination remains the best method to detect occlusal caries in young permanent molars in children, FACE is an effective and accurate diagnostic tool that may aid in detection and treatment decisions.

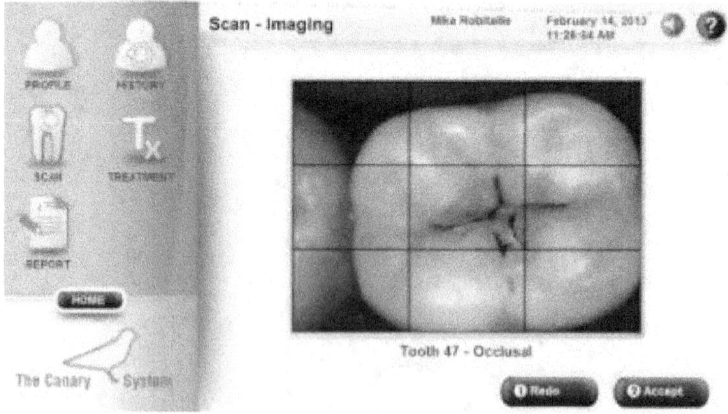

Figure 75 a: Scan Imaging

146

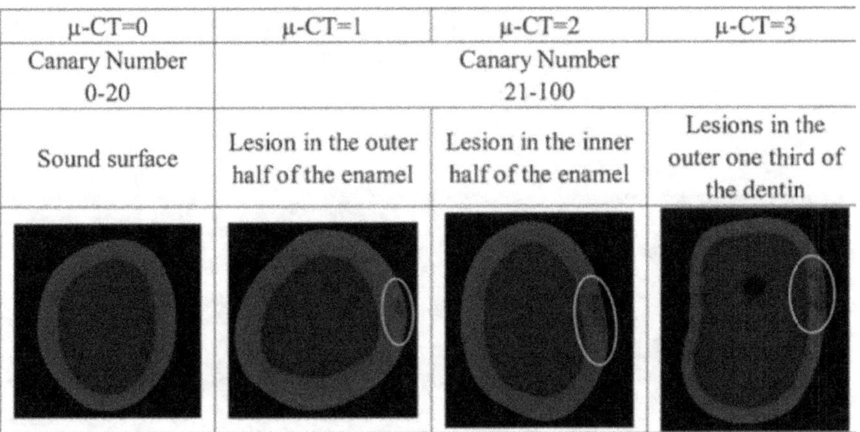

μ-CT=0	μ-CT=1	μ-CT=2	μ-CT=3
Canary Number 0-20	Canary Number 21-100		
Sound surface	Lesion in the outer half of the enamel	Lesion in the inner half of the enamel	Lesions in the outer one third of the dentin

Figure 75 B: Interpretation

This figure represents typical cross-sectional images of μ-CT image for each category. White circle indicates location of caries lesion.

Technology-based caries detection methods, such as Quantitative light-induced fluorescence (QLF), red laser fluorescence device (DIAGNOdent: DD, KaVo, Biberach, Germany), near infrared light transillumination (NILF), and optical coherence tomography (OCT), have been developed in the past years. When detecting approximal enamel and dentinal caries, QLF has comparable performance to the visual inspection and radiography ,DD has better value when de- tecting occlusal caries rather than approximal surfaces ,NILF has similar sensitivity and specificity to DR when detecting non-cavitated approximal caries .OCT can be used in many aspects, e.g. in- dicating tooth demineralization , measuring enamel thickness .monitoring early enamel occlusal caries and lesion progression over time , However, there are no published studies about using OCT to detect non-cavitated approximal caries of posterior teeth, especially with the adjacent teeth existing.

PTR/LUM is another non-invasive, non-ionizing radiation, non-contacting method to detect caries. PTR/LUM value (Canary Number) are calculated from PTR-amplitude response, PTR-phase response, LUM-amplitude response, and LUM-phase response, which measure the reflected heat and light [18]. PTR/LUM value showed good correlation with volume of demineralized tissue and the lesion depth measured with TMR results [20,34] and μ-CT mineral loss measurements [20], when detecting smooth surface and occlusal caries. Based on the manufacturer's instruction, the decay zone (Canary Number: 21–70) indicates lesions with depth of 532 ± 322 μm, and the advanced decay zone (Canary Number: 71–100) indicates lesion depth of 1057 ± 441 μm

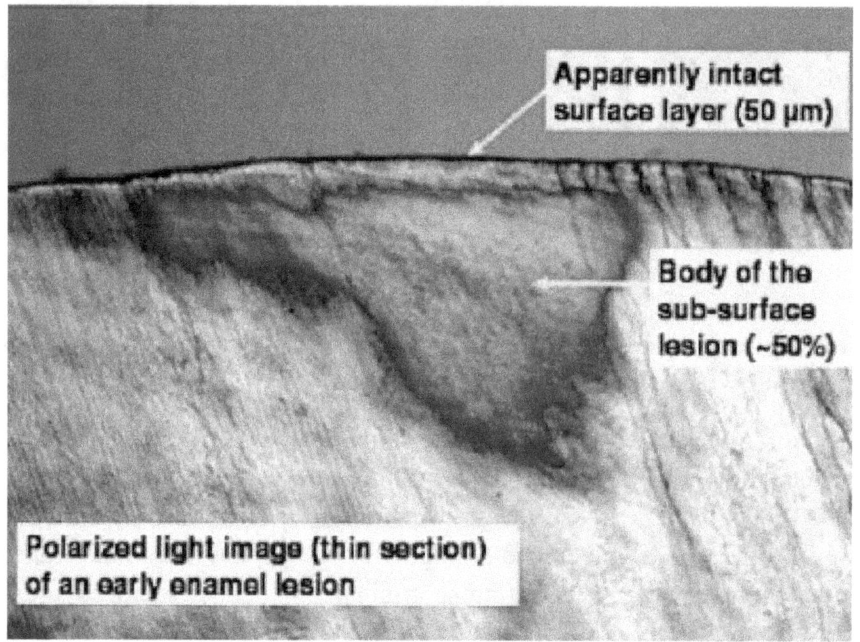

Figure 76: Polarized Light

Cariescan

This device is based on alternating current impedance spectroscopy and involves the passing of an insensitive level of electrical current through the tooth to identify the presence and location of the decay. It is the first dental diagnostic tool to use an impedance spectroscopy to quantify dental caries early enough to enhance preventative treatment. It is not affected by optical factors such as staining or discoloration of the tooth. It provides a qualitative value based on the disease state rather than the optical properties of the tooth.

Bader *et al.* carried out a systematic review comparing CarieScan with a clinical visual examination, bitewing radiograph, and DIAGNOdent reported CarieScan to have superior sensitivity and specificity both 92.5% over other methods.

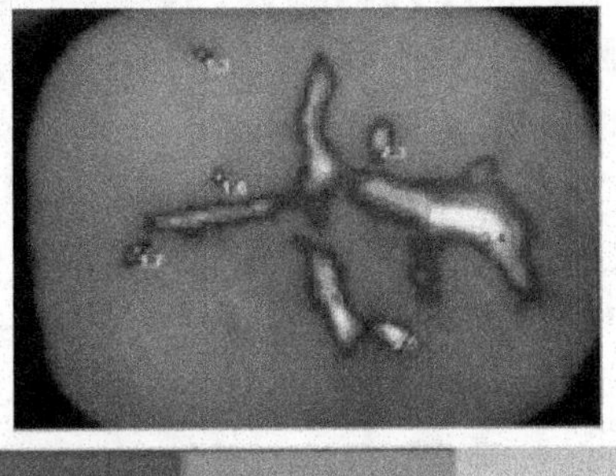

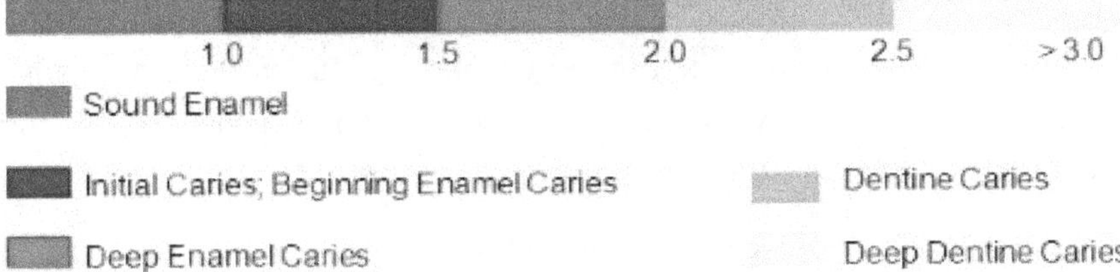

Figure 77: Interpretation

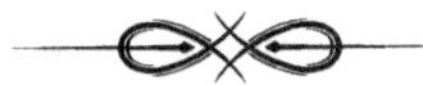

Newer Technologies Include

Spectra Caries Detection Aid

- Spectra is the only caries detection aid that works like Doppler radar to discover caries earlier.

- Early detection means pinpointing problems at an earlier stage, when they traditionally would go undetected. This leads to a more conversative preparation for the filling.

- Spectra uses fluorescence to detect caries in fissures and smooth surfaces that may go unnoticed in X-ray images.

- Carious regions appear yellow to red, while healthy enamel appears green.

- The camera will provide a color as well as a numerical reading showing the depth of the cavity.

- No other caries detection aid can accomplish all of the above.[59]

Multiphoton imaging

Infrared fluorescence

Infrared thermography

Terahertz imaging

Optical coherence tomography

Polarized Raman spectroscopy

Modulated (frequency-domain) infrared photothermal radiometry.

Mechanism of light in detection of dental caries

The regular structure of teeth ensures good propagation of light through the crystalline enamel and tubules of dentin and disruption to structure of a tooth increases likelihood of scattering

- Uptake of fluid into pores created by demineralization in addition to the uptake of exogenous stain, bacterial breakdown products, and other contaminants present as a result of caries process will change the normal interaction of light with tooth structure

- In addition to scattering, these changes will include absorption and fluorescence

- Many of the newer techniques use one or more of these interactions. 17

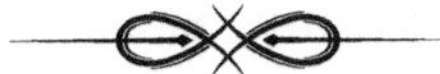

Artificial Intelligence For Caries Detection

Xiao J, Luo J, aimed to use a community-based participatory research strategy to refine and test the usability of an artificial intelligence–powered smartphone app, AICaries, to be used by children's parents/caregivers for dental caries detection in their children.[60]

Previous work has led to the prototype of AICaries, which offers artificial intelligence–powered caries detection using photos of children's teeth taken by the parents' smartphones, interactive caries risk assessment, and personalized education on reducing children's ECC risk. This AICaries study will use a two-step qualitative study design to assess the feedback and usability of the app component and app flow, and whether parents can take photos of children's teeth on their own. Specifically, in step 1, we will conduct individual usability tests among 10 pairs of end users (parents with young children) to facilitate app module modification and fine-tuning using think aloud and instant data analysis strategies. In step 2, we will conduct unmoderated field testing for app feasibility and acceptability among 32 pairs of parents with their young children to assess the usability and acceptability of AICaries, including assessing the number/quality of teeth images taken by the parents for their children and parents' satisfaction.

The study is funded by the National Institute of Dental and Craniofacial Research, United States. This study received institutional review board approval and launched in August 2021. Data collection and analysis are expected to conclude by March 2022 and June 2022, respectively.

The study conducted Using AICaries, parents can use their regular smartphones to take photos of their children's teeth and detect ECC aided by AICaries so that they can actively seek treatment for their children at an early and reversible stage of ECC. Using AICaries, parents can also obtain essential knowledge on reducing their children's caries risk. Data from this study will support a future clinical trial that evaluates the real-world impact of using this smartphone app on early detection and prevention of ECC among low-income children.

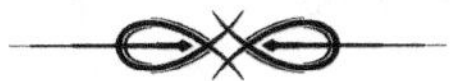

Screening Dental Caries From Oral Photographs

Zhang X, Liang Y, Li W, Liu C, Gu D, Sun W, Miao L. developed and evaluated the performance of a deep learning system based on convolutional neural network (convnet) to detect dental caries from oral photographs.[61]≈

3,932 oral photographs obtained from 625 volunteers with consumer cameras were included for the development and evaluation of the model. A deep ConvNet was developed by adapting from Single Shot MultiBox Detector. The hard negative mining algorithm was applied to automatically train the model. The model was evaluated for: (i) classification accuracy for telling the existence of dental caries from a photograph and (ii) localization accuracy for locations of predicted dental caries.

The system exhibited a classification area under the curve (AUC) of 85.65% (95% confidence interval: 82.48% to 88.71%). The model also achieved an image-wise sensitivity of 81.90%, and a box-wise sensitivity of 64.60% at a high-sensitivity operating point. The hard negative mining algorithm significantly boosted both classification (p < .001) and localization (p < .001) performance of the model by reducing false-positive predictions.

The study concluded deep learning model is promising to detect dental caries on oral photographs captured with consumer cameras. It can be useful for enabling the preliminary and cost-effective screening of dental caries among large populations.

Paxnet: Dental Caries Detection In Panoramic X-Ray Using Ensemble Transfer Learning And Capsule Classifier

Caries lesions are typically diagnosed by radiologists relying only on their visual inspection to detect via dental x-rays. In many cases, dental caries is hard to identify using x-rays and can be misinterpreted as shadows due to different reasons such as low image quality. Hence, developing a decision support system for caries detection has been a topic of interest in recent years.

Arman Haghanifar, Mahdiyar Molahasani Majdabadi, Seok-Bum Ko proposed an automatic diagnosis system to detect dental caries in Panoramic images for the first time, to the best of authors' knowledge. The proposed model benefits from various pretrained deep learning models through transfer learning to extract relevant features from x-rays and uses a capsule network to draw prediction results. On a dataset of 470 Panoramic images used for features extraction, including 240 labeled images for classification, our model achieved an accuracy score of 86.05\% on the test set. The obtained score demonstrates acceptable detection performance and an increase in caries detection speed, as long as the challenges of using Panoramic x-rays of real patients are taken into account. Among images with caries lesions in the test set, our model acquired recall scores of 69.44\% and 90.52\% for mild and severe ones, confirming the fact that severe caries spots are more straightforward to detect and efficient mild caries detection needs a more robust and larger dataset. Considering the novelty of current research study as using Panoramic images, this work is a step towards developing a fully automated efficient decision support system to assist domain experts.

Dayak Onion (Eleutherine Palmifolia (L) MERR) As An Alternative Treatment In Early Detection Of Dental Caries Using Certainty Factor

Dayak onion plants are traditionally used by the Dayak tribe as a medicinal plant to treat dental caries. This plant contains compounds that can inhibit the growth of bacteria that cause dental caries. The public has not yet known about alternative dental caries treatment derived from Dayak onions. This is due to the lack of public knowledge about how to early diagnose dental caries and how to treat using Dayak onions. Expert systems with the Certainty Factor method can be used as a solution in diagnosing early dental caries. The data used in this study consisted of 20 symptoms of dental caries and 6 types of dental caries. This study shows the percentage level of confidence in the results of the initial diagnosis of the type of dental caries suffered by using the certainty factor method and the handling of the diagnosis using the Dayak plant as an initial treatment solution. The results of the accuracy-test showed that the early dental caries diagnosis system was working well.

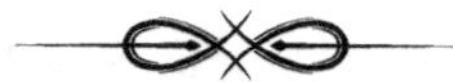

A New Method For Dental Caries Diagnosis Using Convolutional Neural Networks And Bees Algorithm

The diagnosis of dental caries consists of the detection of the lesion followed by its assessment and classification, in terms of the stage of progress and its activity (whether a lesion is active and continues to progress or is arrested and the progress has stopped).[62]

In an attempt to reduce the variability in clinical diagnosis and improve its accuracy, several techniques have been developed for the detection and assessment of occlusal caries. These include fiber optic transillumination, laser or light or infrared fluorescence, electrical resistance and more recently digital radiography, infrared thermography, optical coherence tomography (OCT), tera-hertz imaging and digital photography analysis [7, 8]. The current procedure assumes that the image is recorded on an X-ray film and that it is interpreted by a human expert. Obviously, this suffers from the human error and error with visual inspection, which may further be enhanced by poor quality of the images. Many investigators believe that automation of dental caries screening analysis increases the rate of early detection and diagnosis accuracy. In recent years, machine learning algorithms have been successfully applied on medial signals and images Regarding dental caries, several methods based on artificial neural networks, support vector machine and fuzzy systems have been proposed for dental caries diagnosis.

A class of machine learning techniques named deep learning was developed mainly since 2006, where many layers of non-linear information processing stages or hierarchical architectures are exploited. Deep learning performance is better than the existing classification methods. In the conventional machine learning methods such as multi-layer Perceptron neural network (MLPNN), fuzzy systems and support vector machine (SVM) it is needed to extract the effective features manually . In this context, the convolutional neural networks (CNN) is able to learn the feature vector directly from the training data without any hand-crafting to determine the feature vector .

CNNs are special type of MLP. They are similar to neural networks in the following aspects. They are made up of neurons with weights and biases which have to be learned. Some inputs are given to each neuron. Then, an operation of dot product is performed followed by an optional function of nonlinearity. CNN is buildup of basically three types of main layers. They are Convolutional layer, Pooling layer and a fully connected layer with a rectified linear activation function (ReLU) . The main structure of CNN is shown in Figure 78 .The CNN network can be expanded by adding more convolution and pooling layers. In this figure, CNN has two convolution and pooling layers.

The convolution layer performs feature extraction, and it is usually interspersed with sub-sampling layers to reduce the computation cost. Each layer contains multiple neurons and each of them has their own weights. Feature extraction can be achieved by multiple roll over convolution layers and pooling layers. This is the most important part of the convolutional neural network, and the classification is achieved by the last layer. The convolution layer has a local receptive structure, which is achieved by using a sparse connection, where a neuron with only one part of the input is connected. The sub pooling layer reduces the training difficulty. Furthermore, for each convolution layer neuron, their connection weight is the same, so the computation cost can be significantly reduced. In the convolutional neural network, the pooling layer usually follows the roll accumulation layer, and the pooling layer and the convolution layer may alternately appear many times, thus forming a multi-layer convolutional neural network.

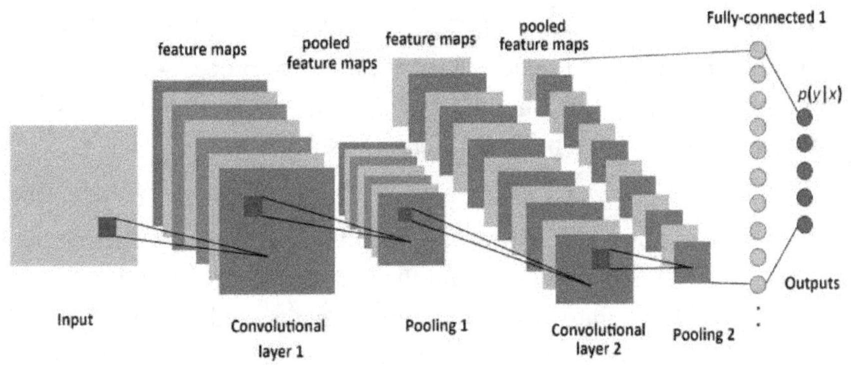

Figure 78: CNN

CNNs were initially used in the area of image processing where it receives raw image pixels on the input end, transform it through a series of hidden layers and finally give the class scores at the other end. Our application is on analyzing signals which are one dimensional, so we use Convolution 1D layers, pooling 1D layers and fully connected layer.

The output of the convolutional layer is given to the pooling (POOL) layer.

Softmax function that gives the probability distribution over each class.Thus, the fully connected layer (FC) will compute the classes which form the final output of the CNN network. Thus the CNN has the architecture of INPUT -CONV - POOL-FC. In summary: A CNN architecture is in the simplest case a list of Layers that transform the input volume into an output volume (e.g. holding the class scores)

There are a few distinct types of Layers (e.g. CONV/POOL/FC are by far the most popular)

Each Layer accepts an input volume and transforms it to an output volume through a differentiable function more detailed by recruiting more bees to follow them than   Each Layer may or may not have parameters (e.g. CONV/FC do, POOL don't) Each Layer may or may not have additional hyperparameters.

The current procedure assumes that the image is recorded on an X-ray film and that it is interpreted by a human expert. Obviously, this suffers from the human error and error with visual inspection, which may further be enhanced by poor quality of the images. This paper proposes an intelligent system based on combination of CNN and BA for dental caries diagnosis. The CNN has performed relatively well on image processing and pattern recognition. The proposed method includes two main modules: classifier module and optimization module. In the classifier module, CNN is used as the main classifier.

In the proposed method, the raw data is fed to CNN layer to extract new features. The features extracted from the convolution and pooling process were broken down into sequential components and fed to the fully connected layer for caries recognition. The caries are classified depending on the output of the fully connected layers. The effective extracted feature in the convolution layer makes the recognition task very easy for fully connected layer.

has good performance in complicated pattern recognition problems, but there are many parameters and hyper-parameters that affect the network's performance significantly. The amount of unknown parameters will increase dramatically with the increase of hidden layer numbers and there are no systematic way to find the optimal value of these unknown parameters and hyper-parameters. To overcome this problem, we have proposed an intelligent method based on BA to find the optimal architecture of the CNN. The main structure of the proposed method is shown in Figure 79.

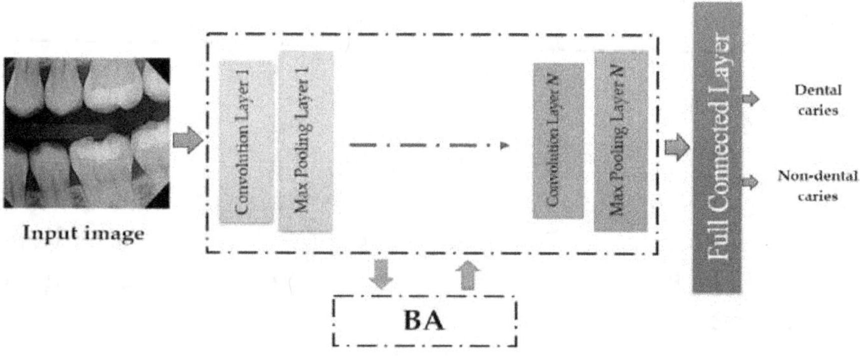

Figure 79: CNN

A study was conducted and the Anonymized periapical radiographic image dataset acquired between March 2017 and October 2018 in the dentistry department of Shahid Beheshti University is used for evaluating the performance of proposed method. All images were clearly revalidated, and dental caries, including enamel and dentinal carious lesions (excluding deciduous teeth), were distinguished from non- dental caries by four calibrated board-certified dentists. The dataset excluded all periapical radiographic images in which the diagnosis of the four examiners did not match, and included the periapical radiographic images for which all four examiners agreed to the diagnosis of dental caries. The dataset consisted of a total of 3000 periapical radiographic images of 778 (25.9%) maxillary premolars, 769 (25.6%) maximally molars, 722 (24.1%) mandibular premolars, and 731 (24.4%) mandibular molars. There were 781 (23.9%) premolars and 772 (25.7%) molars that were diagnosed as dental caries, and 719 (26.1%) premolars and 728 (24.3%) molars diagnosed as non-dental caries. Periapical radiograph images diagnosed as dental caries and non-dental caries were cropped to show only one tooth per image and optimal position. Images were calibrated to standardize contrast between gray/white matter and lesions.

Accurate detection and diagnosis of dental caries reduces the cost of oral health management, and increases the likelihood of natural tooth preservation in the long term. In this study a new method based on intelligent combination of

CCN and BA proposed for automatic diagnosis of dental caries. Several experiments were performed to evaluate the performance of the proposed method and the obtained results showed that the proposed method has better performance in comparison with other methods. The proposed hybrid system of CNN and BA model has delivered promising results as compared to the other conventional studies. In the proposed method, feature extraction and selection techniques are not required.

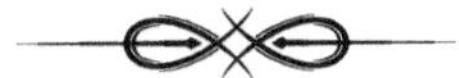

Teledentistry–Based Program For Screening Of Early Childhood Caries In A School Setting

Teledentistry strives to combine telecommunication technology and dental care . The term "teledentistry" was used in 1997, when Cook defined it as "the practice of using video-conferencing technologies to diagnose and provide advice about treatment over a distance ." Telemedicine has a variety of applications in patient care, education, research, administration, and public health along with advantages like ease of access to remote areas, time conservation, and costs of transporting the patient Monitoring home care and ambulatory monitoring of patients can be done using telemedicine .Telemedicine improves communication between health providers who were relatively inaccessible before.

Mainly two types of telehealth programs are practised: 'the store and forward method' and the 'videoconferencing method.' The former is used in case of non-emergency situations when images and information are collected and mailed to the specialist for consultation. This is the most commonly used system in dentistry and has found an effective use for orthodontic consultations. The latter method involves the use of videoconferencing equipment at both locations for a 'real-time' consultation to take place.

The major applications of teledentistry programs have been for specialist referrals and for consultations . There have been previous efforts to use this technology for the diagnosis of pathological conditions . For a long time, dental caries detection has been done by visual and tactile examination. Few studies have evaluated the use of intraoral photographs or digital images for the diagnosis of dental caries . The use of intraoral cameras in the epidemiological setting has been shown to be acceptable to children . An advantage that the use of intraoral photographs has over visual examination methods in such studies is the ability to archive intraoral photographs. This permits multiple scorers to score the images as well as remote scoring and longitudinal analysis .

A program for promoting dental health should be designed such that it is accessible to all, less time-consuming, cost-effective, and cause minimal disruption of daily routines. School-based dental health programs serve most of these criteria, but for the fact that a dentist has to be present physically at school during school hours. The combination of teledentistry programs and school dental health programs could be the ideal answer for overcoming the major barriers to achieving a head start toward oral health care. It is in line with this idea that this study was initiated to assess the reliability and feasibility of using teledentistry for screening and diagnosis of dental caries in children between the age groups of three and six years.

A study was conducted in three different schools in and around Porur, Chennai where the study population consisted of three- to six-year-old healthy school-going children. All children studying in lower kindergarten (LKG), upper kindergarten (UKG), and first standard (Ist Standard) were invited to participate in this study (total of 318). Children within six years of age whose permanent teeth had erupted and children who were uncooperative during the procedure even after behavior modifications were excluded from this study.

This study commenced after a letter of information regarding objective, time, date, and procedure of this study was circulated to the three schools and permission was issued by the respective heads of the institution. Parental consent was obtained for all the children who participated in this study .

The study population (312 children) was divided into three groups as per year of study at school, Group I—students studying in LKG (three- to four-year-olds), Group II—students studying in UKG (four- to five-year-olds), and Group III—students studying in Ist standard (five- to six-year-olds).

Five patients, not related to the study, whose decayed, missing, filled teeth (dmft) was recorded with visual examination and with photographs were used as calibration for the examiner. Examiner 1 and examiner 2 (E1 and E2) examined the patients in person on two separate occasions, 48 hours apart. The calibration was accepted if the results of the measurements at baseline and at 48 hours were the same in more than 90% of the cases.

Similarly, both examiners observed photographs of five patients separately and calculated dmft. The calibration was accepted if the examiners' scores were the same in more than 90% of the cases at baseline and at 48 hours.

Phase I - Gold Standard Phase

This study was conducted in two phases. In phase I, E1 examined the children under the light of the intraoral camera and dmft was noted. E1 also made photographs of the teeth of the each child using a 2.5 megapixel intraoral camera (Dr. Schwartz Home Care Intraoral Camera, Japan). The children were examined in their respective schools. In each quadrant, the molars were photographed separately. The lingual and labial aspects of mandibular and maxillary anteriors were taken separately. A total of eight intraoral images were generated for each patient. A proforma was prepared to collect the data regarding the oral health status and general information. This included information about age, year of study, relevant medical history, and history of previous dental visits.

The index of choice was decayed, missing, filled teeth index (dmft) as all children were in their primary dentition. The index used was the dmft index put forth by Gruebbel AO in 1944, which is the most accepted and used index for primary teeth caries evaluation. A tooth was considered decayed (D) if there was visible evidence of cavitation. This included teeth with untreated dental caries and filled teeth with recurrent caries. Teeth with restorations were scored as filled (F). The missing component (M) included only those teeth lost due to caries. In case of missing anterior teeth, it was ascertained by asking the children if the tooth loss was following trauma or due to caries and scored accordingly by the examiner. All the teeth are scored and the dmft score of a child could range from 0 to 20.

Phase II

The images captured at school were transferred to a computer. Then, E1 examined the images on the computer LCD 15-inch screen with resolution of 1,440 × 900 and scored the teeth for each student. These dmft values were calculated after a washout period of two weeks. The images of the teeth were examined separately by another examiner designated as E2 on the same computer. Three values of dmft index scores were generated for every patient who was screened: dmft1—as examined and scored by E1 in gold standard phase, dmft2—as examined and scored by E1 (Image), and dmft3—as examined and scored by E2 (Image).

The total study population was further divided into three groups, of which 102 children were in Group I (LKG), 106 children were in the Group II (UKG), and 102 children were in Group III (IstStandard).

The extent of dental tissue destruction during the treatment of white spot lesions (WSLs) increases with the severity of the lesion. If the depth and shape of WSLs can be predicted with a non invasive diagnostic method before dental caries treatment, more conservative interventions can be planned. Given the superiority of high-frequency ultrasound (HFUS) imaging in observing the internal structures of the body, the present study aimed to verify the possibility of HFUS imaging to examine the depth and shape of WSLs. We prepared tooth samples and developed a biomicroscopic system with a HFUS transducer to obtain images of normal and WSL regions. HFUS images were compared with conventional ultrasound images and micro–computed tomography images. HFUS distinctly differentiated demineralization within WSL and normal regions. WSL depth calculated in the micro–computed tomography image was similar to that in HFUS. This study revealed that HFUS imaging has the potential to detect early dental caries and offer information on the invasion depth of early dental cari Diagnostic potential of inflammatory biomarkers in early childhood caries - A case control study

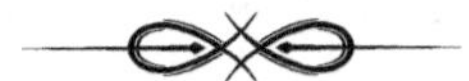

Diagnostic Potential Of Inflammatory Biomarkers In Early Childhood Caries – A Case Control Study

Lvrindasharmaaconducted a non invasive study for diagnosis of dental caries. Optimum sensitivity and specificity for IL -6 , IL-8 and TNF Alpha was observed.[63]

These cytokines might be exploited as a diagnostic and prognostic marker for caries.

The aim of the study was to evaluate salivary levels of inflammatory cytokines in children with ECC to assess their potential as non-invasive biomarkers. 50 subjects were recruited (25 ECC patients and 25 healthy children). Saliva samples were taken from all subjects and collected again from patients after rehabilitative intervention. Levels of IL-6, IL-8 and TNF-α were determined using ELISA. Cytokines level were statistically correlated with each other and with DMF score along with ROC curve analysis. Salivary levels of IL-6, IL-8 & TNF-α were significantly higher in patients which got significantly reduced after rehabilitative intervention. Levels of these cytokines were significantly associated with severity of dental caries. These cytokines were correlating with each other along with DMF score upon Spearman correlation. ROC curve reveals optimum sensitivity and specificity of these cytokines for diagnosis in ECC with absolute levels observed for IL-6.The study concluded significant elevation of IL-6, IL-8 and TNF-α with optimum sensitivity and specificity might imply their involvement as potential non-invasive diagnostic/prognostic markers in ECC.

Systematic Assessment Of Salivary Inflammatory Markers And Dental Caries In Children: An Exploratory Study

Børsting T, Venkatraman V, Fagerhaug TN, Skeie MS, Stafne SN, Feuerherm AJ, Sen A. tried to investigate associations between a wide panel of salivary inflammatory markers and the presence of dental caries among children.[64] In this cross-sectional study, 176 children, aged 7-9, underwent a dental examination. Information on the children's oral health habits and lifestyles was collected from their mothers. In addition, saliva samples were collected and analyzed using a multiplex immunoassay. Of 92 inflammatory markers measured, 56 were included in the statistical analyses. To identify potential inflammatory markers associated with caries, we applied low to advanced statistical analyses. First, we performed traditional logistic regression analysis followed by Bonferroni corrections. Thereafter, a more robust and less conservative statistical approach, i.e. Least Absolute Shrinkage and Selection Operator (LASSO), was applied. The models were adjusted for potential confounders.[64]

Of the 176 children in the study, 22.2% were affected by caries. Among the 56 salivary inflammatory markers, only macrophage colony-stimulating factor 1 (CSF1) was selected by the LASSO and found to be positively associated with the presence of caries. The study concluded an association between CSF1 and the presence of caries may be of clinical value in caries risk management and early diagnosis. Larger studies are warranted to assess the replicability of our findings.

Interleukin-6: A Potential Salivary Biomarker For Dental Caries Progression—A Cross-Sectional Study

Resistance or susceptibility to caries is significantly correlatetd with the alterations in salivary

Proteins and cytokines , a useful biomarker in predicting caries risk and prognosis.

Bacteria colonize the oral cavity and lead to inflammation which induces both innate and adaptive immune response by a host.

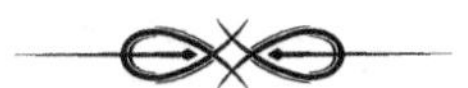

The Impact Of MUC5B Gene On Dental Caries

T Cavallari, H Salomão, ST Moysés, SJ Moysés, RI Werneck et al identified the impact of MUC5B polymorphisms on dental caries. A case–control study was performed with patients recruited at Pontifícia Universidade Católica do Paraná. These individuals were aged 12 years old or more. Dental caries was diagnosed using the International Caries Detection and Assessment System, and the effects of socioeconomic, dietary, and hygiene factors on dental caries were investigated. Buccal cells were collected, and their DNA was extracted and amplified using PCR. Uni-, bi-, and multivariate analyses were performed.[65]

It was seen two hundred patients were recruited, 100 were assigned to the case group and 100 to the control group. In the bivariate analysis, the following variables showed significant results: ethnicity ($p = .008$), biofilm ($p < .001$), and gingivitis ($p < .001$). The MUC5B gene affected dental caries with the markers rs2735733 ($p < .001$), rs2249073 ($p < .001$), and rs2857476 ($p < .001$). In the multivariate analysis, the biofilm variable remained significant ($p = .026$), as did the following markers from the MUC5B gene: rs2735733 ($p = .019$), rs2249073 ($p < .025$), and rs2857476 ($p < .005$).

The study concluded Genetic variations in the MUC5B gene can influence dental caries.

Photoemission Spectra Of Sound Tooth And Those Of Different Carious Stages

Laser-induced fluorescence (LIF) is the optical emission from molecules that have been excited to higher energy levels by absorption of photons. One of the most frequently used applications of LIF is measuring a biological preparation with a dye. A fluorescing dye is chosen which binds to specific structures inside a cell so that when the preparation is lit by a laser, an image of the structures can be made. Sometimes not even a dye is needed but already part of an organism, for example, photosynthesis.

Laura E. Tam, DDS, et al in (2001), reviewed current knowledge concerning conventional and new diagnostic methods for occlusal caries. These methods have several limitations, particularly in their ability to diagnose early carious lesions. Part II examines new and emerging technologies that are being developed for the diagnosis of occlusal decay. Electrical conductance measurements and quantitative laser- or light-induced fluorescence represent

Ana Maria COSTA, Lillian Marley de PAULA, Ana Cristina Barreto BEZER in (2007), evaluated the use of a laser autofluorescence device for detection of occlusal caries in permanent, was found that the laser detection method produced high values of sensitivity (0.93) and specificity (0.75) and a moderate positive predictive value (0.63). The laser device showed the lowest value of likelihood ratio (3.68). Kappa coefficient showed good repeatability for all methods. Although the laser device had an acceptable performance, this equipment should be used as an adjunct method to visual inspection to avoid false positive results .

Anttonen, Vuokko in (2007) used Laser autofluorescence in detecting and monitoring the progression of occlusal dental caries lesions and for screening persons with unfavourable dietary habits This study focused on the clinical use of laser autofluorescence compared to visual inspection (VI) for detecting and monitoring the progress of caries lesions during a one-year follow-up period and for screening subjects with unfavorable dietary habits causing demineralization of teeth .

Roxana Ranga1et al in 2007, has attempted to emphasize the efficiency of laser- autofluorescence (AF) and fibre optic trans-illumination (FOTI) as complementary methods for diagnosing the early caries lesion. It has also demonstrated the interactive and didactic role of the Diagno dent pen.

Bennett T. Amaechia in 2009 described the various technologies available to aid the dental practitioners in detecting dental caries at the earliest stage of its formation, assessing the activities of the detected carious lesion, and quantitatively or qualitatively monitoring of the lesion over time. The need and the importance of these technologies were also discussed. The data discussed are primarily based on published scientific studies and reviews from case reports, clinical trials, and in vitro and in vivo studies.

Fardad Shakibaie, Roy George, L. J. Walsh, in 2011, proposed the principle of the fluorescent phenomenon, then explore the scientific background of fluorescent studies on the dental tissue. The laser-induced fluorescence can be used to detect and diagnose dental caries, calculus and bacterial biofilms in dental applications.

Pini *et al.* used laser fluorescence to detect residual pulp tissue within the root canal, using a 308 nm wavelength ultraviolet laser, while Sarkissian and Le used 366, 405, and 440 nm wavelengths to distinguish remaining pulp tissue and bacteria from normal hard tissue in root canals. Most work using autofluorescence in dentistry has employed visible light as the excitation source

Yao-Sheng Hsieh et al in 2013 described the applications of dental optical coherence tomography (OCT) in oral tissue images, caries, periodontal disease and oral cancer. The background of OCT, including basic theory, system setup, light sources, spatial resolution and system provided. The comparisons between OCT and other clinical oral diagnostic methods are also discussed.

Laser-induced emission was used to distinguish between emission from dental caries and sound tooth and to investigate the relation between emission intensity and the amount of decay.

The spectra were detected with a USB 2000+UV-VIS (PC2000, "Ocean Optics", Inc., Dunedin, FL, USA). A computer was utilised to control the system and to store and show data. The spectra were stored by the spectrometer specialized program (OOI Base, "Ocean Optics", Inc. Dunedin, FL, USA) and were analyzed and graphically represented with another computer program (Origin 5.0, Microcal Software, Inc., Northampton, MA, USA) shwon in Figure 3.

Computer- Aided Radiographic Method (CARM)

Computer- aided radiographic method exploits the measurement potential of computers in assessing and recording lesion size. In the new Trophy 97 system, artificial intelligence software (Logicon caries detector) is integrated: approximal carious lesions are diagnosed and evaluated with the aid of unique histologic database, allowing graphic visualization of the size and progression of the lesion.

At both D1 and D3 thresholds, computer- aided methods offer high levels of sensitivity for approximal lesions. Earlier soft wares paid some trade off high with specificity, but newer methods also have high values for this measure. Wenzel reported that the major advantages may be the significant dose reductions and the ability for image quality manipulation.

Terahertz Pulse Imaging (TPI)

Terahertz pulse imaging (TPI) is s relatively new imaging technique that has been demonstrated in both non-biological applications. Although, the TPI system is a new technique for imaging caries using non ionizing impulses of terahertz radiation, (an electromagnetic radiation) and its ability to detect early stages of caries lesions in various sections of teeth and a hope in future when this technique could indicate caries in all areas of teeth. Terahertz systems are relatively expensive and do not offer the resolving power of radiographic examination. This system also needs more researches to make it possible to be inserted into the mouth for in vivo studies, while it is expected that technological developments will improve the systems to bring them within easy reach of dentists. The coherent detection scheme of system will be safer than those employing X- rays. Unlike radiography TPI also delivers a spectrum of different frequencies for each pixel measured. This offers the possibility of using that spectrum for diagnosis that goes beyond simply measuring mineralization levels.

Pickwell *et al.* compared terahertz pulsed imaging (TPI) with transmission microradiography (TMR) for depth measurement of enamel demineralizations. It was concluded that TPI measured demineralization in the range of 47%.

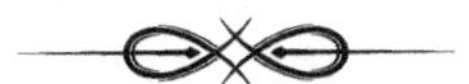

Dermatoglyphics

Dermatoglyphics deals with the study of the epidermal ridges and their configurations on the volar surfaces of fingers, palms, and soles. The volar pads are mound-shaped elevations on each finger above the proximal end on the distal metacarpal bone. The size and position of these pads are responsible for the ridge patterns to an extent

It is the scientific study of dermal ridge configurations on palmar and plantar surfaces of the hands and feet. Dermal ridges and primary palate, both are formed during 6th–7th week of intrauterine life; therefore, hereditary and environmental factors causing changes in fingerprint patterns may also lead to dental anomalies.

A study was conducted with the aim to evaluate and compare the correlation between dermatogly .The study of the human hand has always been fascinating, as the human skin is the largest and delicate organ of the human body that can perform many vital functions in life. The palms of the hands and the soles of the feet are covered with two totally distinct classes of marks. The most conspicuous features are the creases or folds of the skin which interest the followers of palmistry.

These folds or creases could be an indicator of certain congenital abnormalities.

History :

Scientifically, the term palmistry means dermatoglyphics. The term "dermatoglyphics" is coined by **Cummins and Midlo** in 1926. It is derived from the Greek word "Derma" meaning skin and "glyphic" meaning carvings.. Toward the end of the 19th century, Sir Francis Galton, a British anthropologist, began his observations of fingerprints as a mean of identification and put forth a rule called "proof of no change," which states that an individual's dermatoglyphics remain unchanged throughout his/her lifetime. Dermal ridge differentiation takes place in the early stages of fetal development. The ridges are influenced by blood vessel–nerve pairs at the border between the dermis and epidermis during prenatal development. These ridge patterns will get influenced by factors such as inadequate oxygen supply, unusual distribution of sweat glands, and alterations of epithelial growths during the prenatal development.

The ridged skin is considered to be a sensitive indicator of intrauterine dental anomalies because it originates from the same fetal volar pads as that of the teeth and they originate from the same ectodermal layer in the 6th–7th week of embryonic life. Hence, when an intrauterine dermal damage occurs, a tooth anomaly can be expected.

The resulting ridge configurations are genetically determined and influenced or modified by environmental forces. In a similar way, development of dermal ridges and congenital deafness seems to be interlinked as they develop at around the same time.

Herschel was the first to experiment with fingerprints in India.

Schaumann and Alter's (1976) published the book "dermatoglyphics in medical disorders."

Atasu M was the first ones to introduce dermatoglyphics into dentistry.

The possible genetical influence on dental caries is also proved by many researchers. Hans Muhlemann presented a philosophical view when considering the scientific evidence about caries (and periodontal diseases) in humans from the genetic point of view and he concluded that "dental caries is a polyfactorial entity. Could caries not therefore also have a polygenic heritability? One gene could influence the resistance of enamel by determining its chemistry or its morphology; another gene could control the composition of saliva, which could influence partly the oral flora; a third gene could determine eating habits; a fourth could influence one's characteristic personal view of or approach to oral hygiene at home.

Reddy K V *et al* conducted a total of 300 children aged 6–16 years were selected using simple random sampling technique. Their fingerprints were recorded with duplicating ink and caries experience was assessed using International Caries Detection and Assessment System criteria. Chi-square test revealed a significant statistical association between the whorl and loop patterns in caries and caries-free groups. The frequency of whorls was found to be more in caries group and frequency of loops more in caries-free group. Dermatoglyphics could be an effective method as an early and noninvasive and early predictor of dental caries in special children so as to initiate the preventive oral health measures at an early age.[66]

Molecular Fingerprint Imaging To Identify Dental Caries Using Raman Spectroscopy

RAMAN spectroscopy is an analytical method that consists of irradiating a sample with a visible laser source, then determining the type and condition of the substance based of the characteristics of the Raman scattered light that is generated. Evaluations of crystallinity, residual stress analyses, and chemical assessments of molecular structures can thus be performed without contact, damage, or radiation exposure. Since Raman spectroscopy allows analysis at the molecular level without requiring fluorescent probes, fixation, or other types of manipulation, it has recently received attention for its potential applications in several fields of medical science, including dentistry .Various methods of dental analysis using Raman spectroscopy have recently been reported, such as the detection of trace elements in the enamel and the detection of dentin formation in the dental pulp tissue . However, Raman spectroscopy as a means of diagnosing dental caries has long been considered difficult. The reason for this is that the sites of dental caries generate fluorescence noise that exceeds the Raman light and varies according to measurement site and configuration. Recently, however, the combination of Raman spectroscopy with optical coherence tomography and fluorescence subtraction methods using multichannel lock-in detection have also been reported in order to avoid fluorescence interference . Furthermore, modern devices have enabled us to collect Raman data at various measurement sites and configurations and to construct highly reliable algorithms with suitable precision . When such algorithms are used as diagnostic tools, as we have recently reported, Raman spectroscopy can be used as a novel method for the early diagnosis of dental caries . Moreover, Raman spectroscopy allows for the detection of a threshold state of irreversible structural change at the very early stages of tooth enamel demineralization, as caused, for example, by carbonated beverages (e.g., Coca-ColaTM) Based on the technique's confirmed analytical sensitivity, we firmly believe that, in the near future, Raman spectroscopy will allow for a prompt and efficient evaluation of enamel locations that are likely to develop dental caries with high probability.

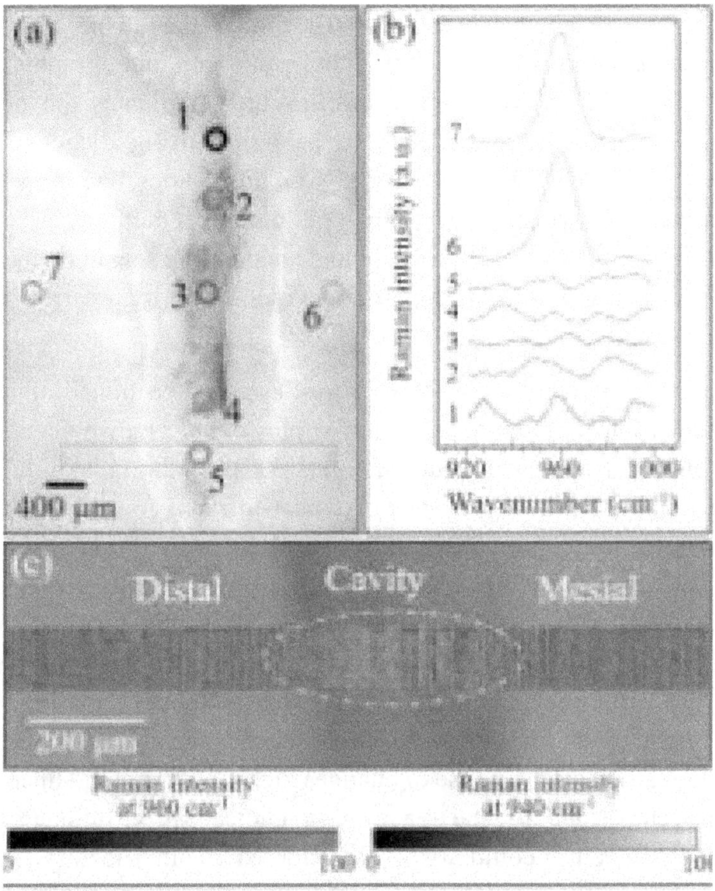

Figure 80: Raman Spectroscopy

To successfully incorporate preemptive medicine into the dental field, highly sensitive diagnostic equipment allowing for the early detection of dental caries will be required. Using Raman spectrophotometry to perform predictive diagnosis with high accuracy (and reliability) at the initial stages prior to the onset of dental caries, and thus intervening before disease development to prevent dental caries, is now technologically possible. In addition, Raman spectrophotometry does not require exposure to radiation. Gonzalez *et al.* have previously reported that, in Japanese subjects, 3.2% of cancers were due to radiation used in medical diagnostic tests .Pearce *et al.* have reported that, among children who have been exposed to radiation used in medical diagnostic tests, the risk of subsequently developing leukemia and brain tumors could reach as much as three times higher than normal. Currently, diagnostic imaging in dentistry consists mostly of bitewing and panoramic radiography as well as CT imaging .Because Raman spectroscopy eliminates the need for radiation exposure, it is believed to be a promising diagnostic tool. Moreover, diagnosis of non-cavitated proximal caries has long been a challenging task when conventional radiographic methods are used . Accordingly, efforts have been made to develop more sensitive diagnostic tools for detecting initial lesions in populations with high caries risk and prevalence.

Among these innovative approaches are the proposed transillumination-based caries detection methods, which employ either a narrow-beam white light , as in fiber-optic transillumination (FOTI) and digital imaging fiber-optic transillumination (DIFOTI), or a near-infrared source , as in near-infrared transillumination (NIRT). Both of these methods are based on the same principle, which exploits the differences in photon scattering/absorption between healthy and disrupted enamel crystals, imaging the latter in dark shadow. Caries detection by laser fluorescence (LF) exploits the semi-empirical finding that a monochromatic red light applied to a tooth location with caries can excite a strong (intrinsic) fluorescence emission because of changes in the tooth tissue. This increase in fluorescence is mainly due to a bacterial photosensitive pigment present in caries tissue, but it could also be contributed by other factors related to oral hygiene. The FOTI/DIFOTI, NIRT, and LF methods have all been commercialized in dentistry, and their caries detection sensitivity/specificity is currently under examination . Nowadays, the LF method is perhaps the most advanced radiation-free method available to enhance early identification of caries and to follow their development through regular successive examinations.

Raman spectroscopy is as an alternative radiation-free method that is superior in sensitivity to LF. We anticipate that the Raman method could play a key diagnostic role in future dentistry now that Raman devices have a sufficiently high sensitivity to be suitable for both diagnostic and preventive purposes.

We have previously established working algorithms for Raman spectrometry in the diagnosis of surface caries in the enamel structure , but its usefulness for caries in the dentin structure has not yet been examined. Dentin, a hard tissue constituting a major component of the tooth, is located between the pulp cavity and the enamel or cementum. The chemical composition of dentin differs greatly from that of enamel, being composed of 70% hydroxyapatite (which makes up 96% of enamel) and 20% collagen fibers. Dentin is softer than enamel; this is believed to be the main reason why dental caries progress rapidly after the dentin is reached. During caries development, when the dentin caries reaches the pulp, severe spontaneous pain may occur as a result of complication by pulpitis. In addition, at that stage of disease development, the dental crown is likely to collapse as a result of the fragility of the tooth, which may ultimately lead to tooth extraction. To avoid this outcome, dental caries must be detected and treated in their very earliest stage, namely, the stage of early enamel demineralization.

Raman spectroscopy helps to visualize and quantify the extent of dental caries buried in the subsurface of the dentin structure. This study is in line with our previous studies of caries in the enamel structure, but this is our first study treating caries that are hardly diagnosable by either visual examination or conventional methods such as X-rays. Applying the method described in this study may help prevent tooth loss and preserve patients' quality of life. Raman photonic diagnostics is the key to the successful application of preemptive medicine in dentistry.

Early Diagnosis And Treatment Of Dental Caries In Pregnancy

Early diagnosis of dental caries in pregnant women is an essential factor in prophylactic and curative therapy in puerperality. Early detection and treatment of dental caries in pregnant women are all the more important if we think that restorative therapy is more expensive and sometimes involves certain risks. The purpose of contemporary dental medicine is to offer practitioners advanced diagnosis techniques in order to objectify dental caries with more than just the help of a dental probe [67]

Clinical examination is beneficial and mandatory only if it is done with great care, thoroughly with non-traumatic fine instrumentation after removing the dental plaque, cleansing, isolating and drying the dental surfaces .

The medical algorithm for early detection of carious lesions requires two basic directions that will allow the correct approach to dental caries therapy:

- evaluation of risk factors with real potential in the appearance of tooth caries, but which did not cause any actual injury;

- early detection of demineralized areas prior to their objectification by clinical and paraclinical examination .

The quantitative detection of dental caries is based on a mandatory clinical examination, along with two other distinct techniques: electrical conductivity and quantitative Light-Induced Fluorescence. More recently, dental radiography and orthopantomography with three-dimensional visualization is considered to be the most effective method of early detection of dental lesions. These methods are able to identify a lesion that has invaded at least half of the thickness of the dental enamel , but unfortunately, they are forbidden during pregnancy.

Advantage of these approaches of identifying primary decalcification lesions – chalky spots – is that these can be treated by remineralization. Electrical conductivity studies are based on the increase of electrical current transmission due to the presence of oral fluid, a good electrical conductor, infiltrated into the porosity of the demineralized or carious enamel. Technically, these measurements can be established by attaching a reference microelectrode, simultaneously with the palpation of the dental surfaces with an intraoral microcamera .

Fluorescent light causes enamel variations that are proportional to mineral deficiency at the dental level, thus facilitating the quantitative assessment of demineralization. The dental surfaces are explored using a device that includes a video camera and the images are obtained, processed and stored by a computer . Three-dimensional image radiography reveals the difference in brightness between normal mineralization areas and those with deficient mineralization or demineralized. By comparing results successively, an assessment of a carious lesion evolution can be accomplished by assessing the immediate study of demineralization, stationary activity or remineralization after therapy. There is a consensus on the clinical principles of differential diagnosis between active, inactive or stationary dental caries .

Determination of oral microbial flora with a cariogenic potential is useful, but not defining for the risk of dental caries. Bacteriological evaluation refers to the presence of lactobacilli and Streptococcus mutans in the bacterial plaque, which are especially found in retention areas (approximal surfaces, fissures and fossas).

Methods for dental caries prophylaxis include a series of measures such as use of fluoride topics, fluoride lacquer and gels, methods which are only applicable for accessible areas. These are especially recommended for children and pregnant women .

Dental caries, being a multifactorial pathology, also involve complex methods of prophylactic and curative treatment such as optimal diet, fighting rickets, correcting dento-maxillary abnormalities and also local prophylaxis.

Pregnancy diet is of great importance in both maintaining general and oral health and fetal development. It has to be calorically efficient, rich in protein, vitamins and mineral salts, and balanced in carbohydrates and lipids .

To reduce the harmful effect of carbohydrates, three rules must be followed:

- carbohydrates are not to be consumed between meals;

- meals are not to be ended with refined carbohydrates;

- teeth hygiene is to be maintained by brushing after each carbohydrate ingestion.

It is advisable to avoid a series of eating habits such as snacking (biscuits, crackers, candies) or consumption of sweet refreshing drinks, because they can generate harmful effects by the carbohydrate composition and by not stimulating the salivary secretion, known to have a buffering capacity beneficial for orodental health .

Saliva plays an indispensable role in protecting against caries and in maintaining oral health. Its constituents maintain and help the repairing of dental enamel, inhibit the growth and multiplication of bacteria and help eliminate food debris.

Far from being an inactive structure in the oral environment, dental enamel undergoes a continuous reshuffle by abrasion, demineralization, restoration and remineralization. Minerals in saliva, especially calcium, and salivary pH are part of the enamel repairing process. Its remodeling may even reduce or remove the chalky white dots in the teeth, which are signs of an incipient cavity .In addition, saliva contains a series of substances that act as a buffer and neutralizes acidity in the dental surfaces and even the oral cavity. Another critical role of saliva is to remove food debris from the external surfaces of the teeth. Salivary flow varies from person to person based on general and local factors. It influences the contact time of food with dental surfaces, as well as the demineralization and remineralization processes.

Salivary flow is increased in mastication and it is affected by the consistency and chemical composition of food. During sleep, the salivary flow is reduced, while the "clearance" of the oral cavity is minimal. For this reason, it is very important to clean the teeth by brushing before bedtime and to avoid food intake after cleaning .

In dental caries prophylaxis in general, and especially in pregnant women, the use of a fluoride- containing mouthwash in the form of sodium or selenium fluoride (sodium or selenium 1-2%) is recommended along with a correct brushing technique. Fluoride-containing chewing gum is a pleasant vector, acting both locally and generally. It stimulates salivary secretion by increasing the interproximal flow. Chewing gum reduces food stores by about 80%, as well as microbial plaque. Varieties containing xylitol reduce the number of Streptococci mutans and also increase the pH of the mouth and bacterial plaque . Investigations, followed by appropriate instrumentation methods, are decisive to the preservation of dental structures. Introduction of fluoridated remineralizing substances contributes to the achievement of contemporary dentistry goals .

Based on these means, dentists and obstetricians are given the opportunity to adopt a model for the early detection and treatment of dental caries with beneficial effects on the oral and systemic health status of pregnant women . The dilemma appears about the decision on how to approach and treat microscopic odontal coronal lesions. Reconstitution therapy is laborious, requires tissue resection imposed by the principles of odontal therapy, is stressful for the pregnant women and is also expensive. In these cases, the remineralization and sealing of fissures and fossets are preferable in pregnancy, being less invasive and much cheaper (8).

During pregnancy, there is a more rapid development of already existing dental caries lesions and thus, a possible aggravation. They often appear in the teeth previously reconstituted by obturations or incrustations, secondary caries and recurrences with brisk evolution and pulp complications. In most cases, the lack or neglect of oral hygiene is at fault..

It has been observed that, at a relatively short time after conception, dentinal hyperesthesia occurs, especially in the cervical area of the teeth, at the erosion, wear or abrasion zones, being triggered by temperature change and sapids (sweet, sour). This is particularly noticeable in the first trimester of pregnancy as a result of vomiting and consumption of acidic foods.

For this reason, it is recommended to rinse one's mouth with mouthwash (Listerine) or 5% bicarbonate solution after each vomit or acidic food ingestion. Special protective shields (bite guard) can also be used along with a gel or fluoridated solutions .

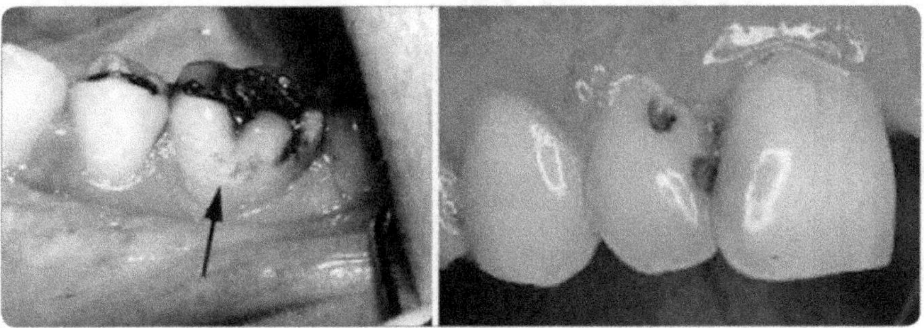

Figure 81: Caries Of Enamel In Pregnant Woman

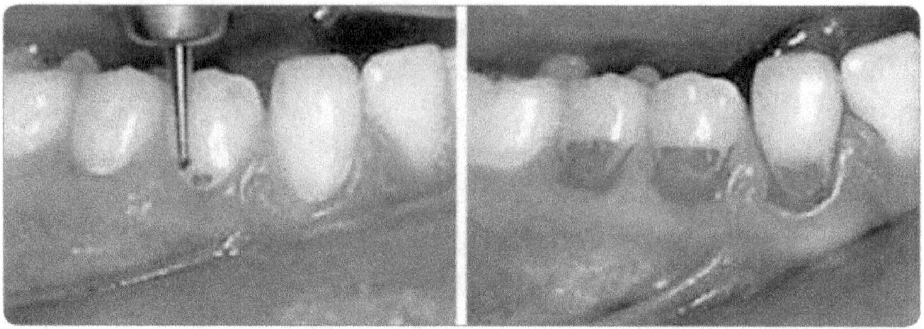

Figure 82: Detection Of Clinical Signs Of Caries

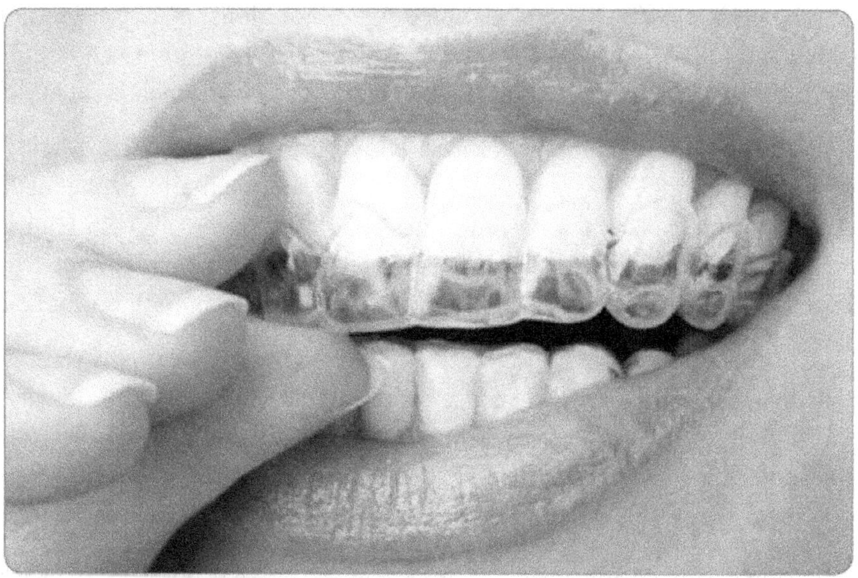

Figure 83: Fluoride Topics, Fluoride Lacquers And Gels To A Pregnant Woman

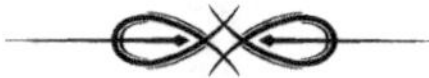

Saliva And Caries

Human saliva contains a large array of proteins, many of which possess a distinct biological function to maintain the homeostasis of the oral cavity system. Alternative splicing and post-translation modifications occurring in the course of gene expression lead to the formation of salivary proteins with various structures. Since Krasnow and Oblatt (Krasnow & Oblatt, 1933) firstly investigated the variation in salivary protein concentration in different individuals, there has been increasing interest in the application of salivary analyses to monitor general health. The National Institute of Dental and Craniofacial Research (NIDCR) started to fund three research groups comprising the Saliva Proteome Consortium in 2004, and they made an effort to identify and catalogue the human saliva proteome including saliva proteins as well as their structurally modified forms (Katsiougiannis & Wong, 2016). With the rapid development of proteomic technology and application of high resolution MS, in-depth proteomic analysis for the salivary protein polymorphisms has recently been achievable (Si, Ao, Wang, Chen, & Zheng, 2015; Sun *et al.*, 2016; Wang, Wang, Wang *et al.*, 2018). These studies revealed the salivary proteome as a sizeable collection of up to 1166 proteins, including 914 in parotid and 917 in submandibular/sublingual saliva (Denny *et al.*, 2008). The majority of these proteins are synthesized and secreted into the oral cavity by the acinar cells of the salivary glands, which can be divided into a few families: proline-rich proteins (PRPs), salivary mucins, salivary α-amylase, salivary cystatins, histatins (small cationic histidine-rich peptides), and statherin and P B peptide (Amado, Lobo, Domingues, Duarte, & Vitorino, 2010; Cabras *et al.*, 2014; Gonzalez-Begne *et al.*, 2009; Zhang, Sun, Wang, & Wang, 2013). The above findings have promoted the gaining of knowledge regarding the association between salivary protein composition and human health, and also provided a promising result in utilizing saliva to explore biomarkers for diagnosis purposes. The noninvasive and simple nature of saliva collection made it interesting to be used for the early diagnosis and risk assessment of a variety of oral diseases, such as Sjögren's syndrome, oral squamous cell carcinoma, periodontitis, and dental caries (Gallo *et al.*, 2016; Hall *et al.*, 2017; Nomura *et al.*, 2012; Wang, Wang, Wang *et al.*, 2018). With an expectedly increasing number of salivary protein species to be identified in the near future, now is the time to devote more attention to the comprehension of their function and to the application of their clinical practice.

Dental caries is one of the most common chronic diseases afflicting a large proportion of the world's population, involved in interactions between the tooth structure, the microbial biofilm formed on the tooth surface, as well as genetic influences and salivary function (Petersen, 2003; Pitts *et al.*, 2017). Saliva contains a variety of proteins participating in maintaining the tooth integrity and preventing caries through several mechanisms: I) formation of acquired enamel pellicle to continuously protect against tooth wear (mucins and proline-rich glycoprotein); II) inhibition of demineralization of exposed tooth surfaces (mucins); III) promotion of enamel remineralization by attracting calcium ions (proline-rich proteins and statherin); IV) antimicrobial activities including prevention of cariogenic species adherence onto enamel surface (histatins and cystatins), microorganism aggregation and clearance from the oral cavity (agglutinin and immunoglobulins), and the secretion of antimicrobial peptides (AMPs) (Gao, Jiang, Koh, & Hsu, 2016; Guo & Shi, 2013; Van Nieuw Amerongen, Bolscher, & Veerman, 2004). Currently, the biological functions of salivary proteins have been extensively studied for their possible relevance to caries risk assessment. For example, low levels of statherin and truncated cystatin S in saliva are found to be associated with caries susceptibility (Rudney, Staikov, & Johnson, 2009). This enhances knowledge of the structure-function relationship of salivary proteins, making it possible to identify potential biomarkers for dental caries, and further to design small, biologically active peptides as instruments to fight against caries, as well as restore functionality in patients in whom the natural protection is compromised.

(1) the protective function of major salivary proteins in cariology; (2) the identification of salivary proteins utilized as biomarkers for caries risk

assessment; (3) bioactive peptides derived from salivary proteins for the therapeutic use against dental caries.

Protective Functions Of Salivary Proteins And Their Potentials As Biomarkers For Caries Risk Assessment

Saliva contains a large number of secreted proteins, including major salivary glycoproteins (proline-rich proteins, mucins and immunoglobulins), minor salivary proteins (cystatins, lysozyme, lactoferrin, agglutinin, and amylase), AMPs (histatins, cathelicidin peptide LL-37, alpha-defensins, and beta-defensins), statherin and P-B peptide, which protect the tooth integrity through either against losing calcium and phosphate ions from the enamel surface or playing antimicrobial role directly .

Therapeutic Anti-Caries Effects Of Bioactive Peptides Derived From Salivary Proteins

A goal of modern dentistry is the non-invasive management of non-cavitated caries lesions involving antimicrobial and remineralization systems in an attempt to prevent disease progress. The study of peptides descended from salivary proteins as a new class of therapeutic agents against dental caries has attracted considerable interest in many research centers Insight into the mechanism of action, in addition to knowledge of the structure-function relationship of salivary proteins and

Surgical oncology :A malignant tumor of the salivary gland often requires surgical treatment. Surgery could involve removing a portion and/or the entire major salivary gland; this reduces salivary flow and may increase the risk of dental caries, as saliva serves the purpose of flushing the oral cavity and also imparts host immunity.

Radiation oncology:

Radiation therapy affects the tissues of oral tissues in several manners. The early changes following radiation therapy include mucositis, atrophy, thinning of the oral mucosa, fibrotic changes, and taste disorders following the atrophy of taste buds. The significant changes involve radiation caries. The term "radiation caries" represents a severe form of rampant caries. Dental caries following radiation therapy mostly results from hyposalivation, which is due to fibrotic changes in major salivary glands.

The most characteristic features of radiation caries are the involvement of tooth at gum level and cusp tip in contrast to normal cavitation, which mostly affects smooth surfaces. The rate of progression of radiation caries is much faster than normal cavitation.

Studies and Trials:

Dental caries has received extensive study. Several studies have sought to find the initiating cause and halt the process. Recently, more sophisticated studies like genomic studies, molecular dynamics studies of polysaccharide carriers based on starch in dental caries, an association of risk factors of dental caries, and polymorphism of the MBL2 gene in *S. mutans* and human clinical trials on dental caries vaccine are a focus of current research. The most recent study looked at bisphenol A glycidyl methacrylate (bis-GMA), which is released into the oral environment from leaching of dental composite and can lead to secondary caries at a margin of restoration.

Treatment Planning for a disease to be treated is a step-by-step process of decision-making or the formation of a protocol. Levels of prevention can classify treatment for dental caries. A widely used taxonomy of prevention describes primary, secondary, and tertiary prevention. These terms can be applied to the disease process of dental caries and can help providers to understand where in the process they can intervene and how they can do so.

Primary prevention is the prevention of the disease process before it begins. Primary prevention would encompass assessing the risk for dental caries and instituting efforts to decrease or remove that risk.

Secondary prevention refers to detecting the presence of the disease early in the disease process and intervening to prevent further development of the disease. For the dentist, this would involve recognizing the signs of the early stages of dental caries, intervening, or referring for intervention.

Tertiary prevention refers to alleviating the effects of the disease and lies primarily within the surgical realm of the dental professional in rehabilitating the damaged tooth. For proper treatment, the international caries classification and management system (ICCMS) has been given, which is a set of clinical protocols such as diagnostic, preventive, and restorative decisions that are necessary to rebuild and restore the tooth structure only when necessary.

As prevention strategies of dental caries may have a relevant impact on avoiding further development of dental caries after restoration, several factors should be considered before implementation of preventive or restorative strategies like past caries experience, oral hygiene status, calculus deposits, and snacking level salivary flow.

Meticulous Maintenance of Oral Hygiene: As dental caries cannot progress without the presence of microorganisms present in dental plaque, daily removal of dental plaque with tooth brushing and flossing is considered to be the best preventive method.

Topical Fluoride Application: Fluoride inhibits dental caries by inhibiting demineralization and enhancing remineralization of tooth structure by the formation of acid-resistant fluorapatite crystal. Various methods that incorporate fluoride in daily life include fluoridated water supply, use of fluoridated toothpaste, use fluoridated mouth rinse, and application of different professional fluoride gels and varnishes.

Application of Pit and Fissure Sealants: Pits and fissures pose non-cleansable morphology and hence are the most susceptible site for the initial development of caries. Application of the pit and fissure sealants leads to the formation of a mechanical barrier that leads to deprivation of nutrition for underlying microbes and hence halts the progression of dental caries.

Xylitol: The main dietary culprit in the formation of dental caries is sucrose. Nowadays, sucrose is getting replaced by xylitol, an artificial sweetener that is not only non-cariogenic but also anti-cariogenic. The possible mechanism of anticariogenicity is the prevention of binding of sucrose to *S. mutans* and the prevention of adhesion of mutans to each other.

Vaccine: As dental caries is an infectious microbiologic disease, continuous attempts have been made to develop an anti-carious vaccine, but to date, none of the vaccines has appeared successful.

Complications:

If dental caries is left untreated for a more extended period, it may lead to several complications based on the nature of the carious lesion. Starting from the small inactive white spot lesion, it may lead to osteomyelitis. Dental caries course through various stages and its progression depends upon the host response and chronicity of the lesion. If the host immune response is weak, dental caries may result in inflammation of the pulp leading to:

- Apical periodontitis
- Periapical abscess
- Periapical granuloma
- Periapical cyst
- Cellulitis
- Abscess
- Periostitis
- Osteomyelitis

Dental caries is not life-threatening, but if the infection spreads through facial planes, patients are at increased risk of sepsis, airway compromise (Ludwig angina), and odontogenic infections, which in one study accounted for 49.1% cases of deep neck abscesses.

Patient education:

The decline of dental caries has been ascribed to several factors. Among all the factors, patient education plays a key role. The patient-related factors include oral hygiene maintenance, reduction in sugar consumption, effective use of fluorides, and routine oral checkup. Patients should be educated to perform regular tooth brushing with fluoridated toothpaste and dental flossing. As sugar consumption is one of the primary etiological factors for dental caries, it is necessary to evaluate the dietary habits of the patient. Patients should be advised to restrict the consumption of sugar-based snacks and drinks to reestablish the balance between demineralization and remineralization.

Caries Mechanism And Its Application To Caries Risk Assessment And Caries Management

The demineralization in dental caries can be inhibited by salivary components, antibacterial agents, and fluoride or reversed by remineralization that requires calcium, phosphate, and fluoride. Progression or reversal of dental caries was driven by the "caries balance," namely, the balance between the pathological factors, primarily (1) cariogenic bacteria, (2) fermentable carbohydrates, and (3) salivary dysfunction, and protective factors, primarily (1) sufficient saliva; (2) remineralization that requires calcium, phosphate, and fluoride; and (3) antibacterial agents.

The Caries Management By Risk Assessment (CAMBRA) philosophy was developed in California following 2 consensus conferences (Featherstone *et al.* 2003, 2007). The newly designed caries risk assessment form was piloted in several dental schools. UCSF and University of the Pacific implemented particularly comprehensive, large-scale pilots, starting in 2003. The forms and procedures were modified over time, and the modified versions were published in the California Dental Association Journal in 2007 **(Featherstone *et al.* 2007; Jenson *et al.* 2007) in** 2 special issues .

Summary :

1. Take dental and medical history.

2. Conduct clinical examination.

3. Detect caries lesions early enough to reverse or prevent progression.

4. Assess the caries risk as low, high, moderate, or extreme using data from 1, 2, and 3 and a short questionnaire.

5. Produce a treatment plan that includes chemical therapy appropriate to the caries risk level.

6. Use chemical therapy that includes fluoride and/or antibacterial agents based on risk level.

7. Use minimally invasive restorative procedures to conserve tooth structure and function.

8. Recall and review at intervals appropriate to the caries risk status.

9. Reassess caries risk level at recall and modify the treatment plan as necessary.

Caries Risk Assessment Procedure Development and Validation

Outcomes studies specifically related to the predictive validity of the caries risk assessment form were conducted and published in 2006 and 2011 (Doméjean-Orliaguet *et al.* 2006; Doméjean *et al.* 2011). As a result of these outcomes studies, the items used in the caries risk assessment for patients aged 6 y through adult were grouped into (1) disease indicators (clinical observations), (2) biological risk factors (expanded to pathological factors), and (3) protective factors. The number of patient records used was 2,351 in the 2006 study and 12,954 in the 2011 study.

The caries risk level was determined by the individual providers based on an assessment of the balance between the disease indicators, the risk factors, and the protective factors, as per detailed instructions previously published (Featherstone *et al.* 2007). Risk levels were assigned as low, moderate, high, or extreme. Extreme was defined as high risk plus hyposalivation, as assessed by visual inspection, medical history, and, if in doubt, measurement of salivary flow rate. Our outcomes studies showed that in our clinics, approximately 5% of our patients are at extreme risk (**Doméjean** *et al.* 2011).

An example of a patient at extreme risk would be the following:

*   **Disease indicators:** Visible cavity, numerous approximal lesions by radiograph, numerous restorations in the past 3 y.

*   **Biological risk factors:** Visible heavy plaque on the teeth, frequent snacking, inadequate saliva flow by measurement and signs of dry mouth, more than 1 medication that has hyposalivatory side effects.

*   **Protective factors:** Once-daily fluoride toothpaste use.

In this case, the assessment would be 7 disease indicators and pathological factors, including hyposalivation and only 1 protective factor, leading to a definite extreme risk patient assessment.

One recent modification to the caries risk assessment (CRA) form clarifies the item about recent restorations. For new patients (6 y through adult), we use "restorations in the past 3 years," whereas for patients of record, we use "new caries-related restorations in the past 12 months." This allows the compliant patient to get "out of the penalty box" in that a patient under continuing care is not relegated to high-risk status for 3 y following restoration placement if the balance of risk and protective factors is otherwise favorable. The fact that caries risk level can be lowered with behavior change and therapeutic intervention may be motivating for patients. The feasibility of lowering caries risk was illustrated in a practice-based research study reported by Rechmann *et al.*, as reported in the present publication (Rechmann *et al.* 2017), where the authors demonstrated dramatic reductions in caries risk status within 18 to 24 mo.

A second CAMBRA caries risk assessment tool (Ramos-Gomez *et al.* 2007) was developed in parallel with the age 6 y to adult form for use with young children aged 0 to 5 y. This form was introduced in the UCSF postgraduate pediatric teaching clinics in 2009. An outcomes assessment was conducted (Chaffee *et al.* 2016) to assess the predictive validity of this additional CRA tool. Very few extreme-risk children were identified, so this assessment was confined to low-, moderate-, and high-risk patients. VAs was the case with older patients, approximately 70% of patients assessed as high risk had new decay at follow-up visits.

Caries Management Outcomes:

A central tenant of CAMBRA is that patient risk assessment levels dictate appropriate, patient-tailored noninvasive therapy: the most intensive preventive interventions are targeted at high-risk and extreme-risk patients, delaying or preventing decay and restorative treatment needs.

Over the first decade of CAMBRA implementation at UCSF, we had accumulated meaningful data on caries risk assessment and caries management based on risk assessment. The age 6 to adult multicomponent CAMBRA caries risk assessment tool, described above, was confirmed as strongly associated with future treatment needs (Chaffee *et al.* 2015a), and the first CAMBRA clinical trial had yielded promising results (Featherstone *et al.* 2012). Less information was available regarding the effectiveness of risk-based caries management in practice. We recently conducted an outcomes assessment (Chaffee *et al.* 2015b) based on patient records for 18,004 eligible patients from 2007 to 2012 in our predoctoral teaching clinic. Caries risk assessment was conducted at baseline as a routine part of clinical care using the CRA methodology summarized above (Featherstone *et al.* 2007). At their initial visit, 11,900 adult patients were assessed as high risk by student providers under the supervision of faculty dentists. Of these patients 2,724 were examined at follow-up after an average of 18 mo.

The recommended chemical therapy for these high-caries-risk patients consisted of (1) fluoride varnish at the initial visit, (2) twice-daily use of prescription fluoride toothpaste (5,000 ppm F), (3) chlorhexidine gluconate 0.12% mouthrinse (once daily for 1 wk every month), and (4) xylitol gum or mints daily. All patients were offered this therapy, but many opted not to receive or use the anticaries products.

To assess the efficacy of the regimen, caries outcomes in 3 patient groups were compared, namely, (1) never received the anticaries products (n = 1,501), (2) took the products once and never returned for refills (n = 900), (3) took the anticaries products and returned at least once for more (n = 323). Although this was a retrospective study and not a controlled randomized clinical trial, these 3 groups provide evidence whether or not the regimen worked to reduce caries increment.

Lesser DFT increment represents a major change in caries increment for a university clinic that serves a largely high-caries, mostly poorly compliant, mostly low socioeconomic status population.

A subgroup of these patients was on a public assistance program, and their products were available at no cost to them. Even then, many did not accept or use the anticaries products, or took them only once, which presumably indicated they did not use them regularly. Comparing the same 3 groupings of none, 1, and 2 or more times, the group that took the products twice or more had 38% lower DFT increment than the group that never received the products. However, because of relatively small numbers (n = 335, 238, and 167, respectively, for the 3 groups), this difference was not statistically significant.

Rechmann *et al.* 2017 conducted study on 18 private practices, 3 community clinics, and 460 patients, each patient followed for up to 2 y. Marked reductions in caries risk status were observed.

The evidence for the CAMBRA approach includes the 2 randomized, controlled, clinical trials summarized above as well as several outcomes studies involving thousands of patients. In the ideal world, further randomized clinical trials should be conducted that include other possible chemical therapeutic regimens, perhaps with lower dropout rates and pediatric participants as well as adults. However, it is very challenging to get funding for such studies that are expensive and take several years to conduct.

Caries Risk Assessment Tools

The CAMBRA (Caries Management by Risk Assessment) CRA procedure for the age group 6 year through adult (Featherstone *et al.* 2007) was developed over a period of years and followed the suggestions of a consensus conference. These CRA procedures have been used in the predoctoral teaching clinics at UCSF for 14 y, and several outcome studies have been conducted (Doméjean-Orliaguet *et al.* 2006; Doméjean *et al.* 2011; Chaffee *et al.* 2015a). These 3 outcomes assessments, each on different cohorts of thousands of patients, demonstrated a clear relationship between CAMBRA-CRA risk levels of low, moderate, high, and extreme with cavitation or lesions into dentin (by radiograph) at follow-up. This risk prediction tool has been updated with time and is now routinely used in these clinics as part of normal clinical practice. The CAMBRA-CRA tool for 0- to 5-y-olds (Ramos-Gomez *et al.* 2007) has demonstrated similar predictive validity (Chaffee *et al.* 2016) and is in routine use in the UCSF postgraduate pediatric dentistry clinics. These CRA tools can be used with confidence. Additions and modifications should not be made unless there is evidence to support such changes.

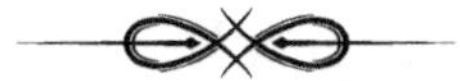

Caries Activity Test

Caries Diagnostic Advances

1) Cariostat Test (Caries Risk Test)

- A new, quick and effective caries activity test.

- CRT has two components:

  a) CRT bacteria – which allows estimation of a number of cariogenic bacteria in the patient's saliva

  b) CRT buffer – which determines the buffering capacity of the same.[68]

CRT bacteria is a two-in-one dip-in-slide test which identifies counts of

a) Mutans Streptococci

b) Lactobacilli

Stimulated saliva is collected and applied to both the sides of the dip-in-slide. Then it is incubated for hrs at 37 0C. The CRT buffer is available in a strip form, which changes color to indicate whether the patient has a high, medium or low buffering capacity. This occurs within five minutes.

2) CariScreen an easy 1 minute test

The quick and easy CariScreen test determines the level of decay-causing bacteria. It takes only one minute to determine if a patient is at low, moderate, or high risk of developing cavities in the future.

Principle:

When adenosine triphosphate (ATP) is brought into contact with the unique liquid-stable luciferase/luciferin reagent within the CariScreen Swab sampling device, light is emitted in direct proportion to the amount of ATP present. The CariScreen meter measures the amount of light generated and provides information as to the level of contamination within seconds.

3) CariFree (Oral BioTech, Albany, OR) is a caries risk assessment and treatment model based on the CAMBRA approach. Caries risk is determined based on a questionnaire and a chair-side measurement of the adenosine triphosphate (ATP) bioluminescence (CariScreen Caries Susceptibility Testing) from the plaque present on specific sites within the oral cavity. The ATP-driven bioluminescence assays have long been used as a quantitative measure of microbial numbers in the packaged food industry and more recently for measuring total bacterial mass in dental plaque. Based on the level of caries risk, the patient is placed on a treatment regimen. This do-at-home treatment includes oral rinses, toothpaste substitutes and chewing gum containing the benefits of xylitol, fluoride and pH neutralizing agents. These specific agents help to modify the salivary environment and build resistance against acid attack. The CariScreen Caries Susceptibility Testing meter can be used chair side and is a validated tool measured instead of the amount of calcium dissolved

The patients will know their test results from the Cari Screen meter within 1 minute. Should their test suggest a moderate to high risk of caries caused by cariogenic biofilm, the dental assistant or hygienist can explain the consequences of a biofilm infection — and the ease and cost-effectiveness of treatment.

Since risk factors change over time, it is recommended that patients take the Cari Screen test once per year. For the most accurate test results, ask your patients to not eat or brush their teeth for at least one hour prior to the test

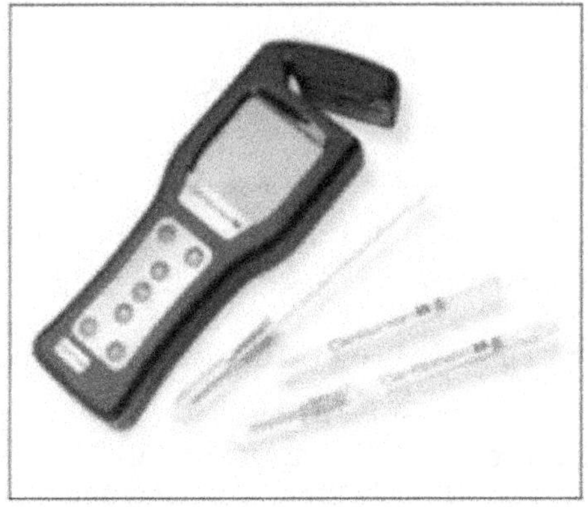

Figure 83: Caries Susceptibility Testing Meter

1	Lactobacillus count test		
		No. of organism	Degree of caries activity
		0-1,000	None
		< 10,000	Slight
		< 1,00,000	Moderate
		< 1,000,000	Marked
2	Dentocult lactobacilli test	> 10,000 C.F.U-high caries activity	
		< 1000 C.F.U-low caries activity	
3	Swab test	pH	Degree of caries activity
		< 4.1	Marked caries activity
		4.2-4.6	Active
		4.5-4.6	Slightiy active
		> 4.6	Caries active

4	Snyder test	24 hrs	48 hrs	72 hrs
		If yellow	If yellow	If yellow
		Marked caries susceptibility	Definite caries susceptibility	Limited caries susceptibility
		If green	If green	If green
		Continue to incubate & observe at 48 hrs	Continue to incubate & observe at 72 hrs	Caries inactive

5	Streptococcus mutans	> 1,00,000/ml of s.mutans in saliva indicate high caries risk
6	Albans test	Change of colour from bluish green (pH 5) to definite yellow (pH < 4) indicates high risk caries

7	Salivary reductase test	Colour	Time (min)	Score	Caries activity
		Blue	15	1	Non conducive
		Orchid	15	2	Slight
		Red	15	3	Moderate
		Red	Immediately	4	High
		Pink/white	Immediately	5	Extreme
8	Fosdick calcium dissolution test	Amount of calcium dissolution is directly proportional to caries activity			

Table 19: Caries Activity Test

Methods	Principle	Uses
Antigen-Specific assays	- Utilize highly specific monoclonal anti-bodies, giving absolute specificity for bacteria of choice	- Includes immunoflorescence, flow cytometry, latex agglutination, immunoblots & solid phase immunoa-ssays
GC-Saliva check SM^{TM}	- Uses a combination of 3 highly specific anti-S.mutans monoclonal antibodies (SWLA-1,2,&3) (17,18) to inc-rease binding & reduce	- Used particularly in tracking transfer of MS from mother to infant, to detect risk of early childhood caries

Table 20: Latest Caries Activity Test

Oratest, a caries activity test was performed on 48 school going children of Mangalore city to estimate efficacy of the test. High statistical significance was found when the means of control and test group were compared [γ = 0.913]. The Oratest is found to be a simple chair side, less time consuming and inexpensive caries activity test.[69]

Lee HS, Lee ES, Kang SM, Lee JH, Choi HJ, Kim BI in 2016 assessed the validity of a new caries activity test that uses dental plaque acidogenicity in children with deciduous dentition.Ninety-two children under the age of three years old underwent clinical examination using the dft index and examinations with two caries activity tests. Plaque samples for the new Cariview(®) test and the saliva sample for the conventional Dentocult SM(®) test were collected, incubated, and scored according to each manufacturers' instruction.

The mean dft index of all of the subjects was 4.73, and 17.4% of the subjects were caries-free. The levels of caries risk based on the new Cariview test score significantly increased with the caries experience (p < 0.01). The test results revealed a stronger correlation with caries indices (dft and dt index) than the conventional SM colony counting method (r = 0.43, r = 0.39, p < 0.01). The study concluded new caries activity test to analyse the acidogenic potential of whole microorganisms from dental plaques can be used to evaluate caries risk in children with deciduous teeth.[70]

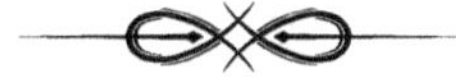

Conclusion

The shift in treatment philosophy from "extension for prevention" to "minimally invasive dentistry" has afforded the dentist the opportunity to diagnosis and manage caries at an early stage.

Caries detection tools aim in early detection of caries and prevents the progression of caries from demineralization to cavitation and its seen None of the mentioned techniques alone are sufficient for diagnosis of dental caries and to be stated as ideal. An ideal caries detection method should capture the whole continuum of caries process.

New devices do offer promise in the monitoring of early incipient lesions of caries, and therefore preventive dentistry techniques may be more appropriately targeted and assessed.

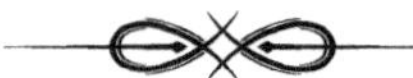

Summary

Test	Characteristics	Intended Use In Clinical Pathway	Other Information
Visual or visual-tactile examination	Identifying caries according to their visual appearance, aided by a dental mirror and probe, on clean and dry teeth	The fundamental step in the detection of caries, but limited in the diagnosis of early lesions. All patients presenting to a dental clinician will receive a visual examination	**Advantages:** completed and interpreted quickly with minimal invasion and little cost except clinician training and time **Disadvantages:** early caries are difficult to observe visually, depth and severity of lesions cannot be assessed, approximal lesions cannot be seen
Radiography	Bite-wing radiology is the most commonly used method. Others include:	Widely used as an adjunct to aid detection and in particular to inform the clinician of the depth and severity	**Advantages:** radiographs aid the detection of caries and are shown to be more sensitive than visual

| | subtraction radiographs which provides a semi-automated method for monitoring progression of lesions (Ellwood 1997; Wenze l 2000) and cone beam computed technology (CBCT) which provides a 3-dimensional image which appears to offer great potential for diagnosis with increased levels of radiation (Horner 2009) | of lesion (Wenzel 1995; Whaites 2013)

 Relevant on occlusal surfaces but also in approximal location which are otherwise difficult to assess visually | examination on approximal and occlusal lesions (Wenzel 2004)
 Disadvantages: l imitations exist when detecting early caries in enamel surfaces. There is a small but real risk over patient exposure to ionizing radiation, which has to be balanced with the patient's age, caries risk and time since previous radiograph (Pitts 2017). Digital radiographic methods have shown benefits for patients with the speed in which they can be viewed and for the ability to manipulate images for increased clarity (Wenzel 2006) |
| Fluorescence | The breakdown | Potential to aid the clinician in | **Advantages:** the potential to |

	of enamel alters the characteristics of its structure, when exposed to light-inducing fluorescence diseased teeth respond differently to sound teeth. There is potential for mineral loss to be quantified and used to aid the diagnostic decision and treatment pathway (Angmar-Månsson 2001; Matos 2011). Fluorescence is typically divided into laser fluorescence and light fluorescence (i.e.	identifying early caries which may not be possible with a visual examination alone. Quantitative light-induced fluorescence (QLF) emits either green or red light and may ascertain whether the lesion is active or arrested	identify changes in tooth characteristics that are otherwise unobservable in a visual-tactile examination **Disadvantages:** uncertainty of the reliability of devices and the ability to detect disease and health

	Diagnodent type devices and QLF type devices)		
Fibre-optic transillumination	Fibre-optic transillumination (FOTI) uses a light emitted from a hand held device which when placed directly onto the tooth illuminates the tooth (Pretty 2006). Any demineralisation should appear as shadows in the tooth due to the disruption of the tooth's structure due to caries	An adjunct to the visual examination, particularly useful for identifying detecting approximal caries, with its strength being in identifying early caries in enamel and dentine (Davies 2001). A further advancement with fibre-optic techniques combines this with a camera to capture an image which may or may not be linked to software for analysis, Digital Imaging FOTI (DIFOTI)	**Advantages:** the potential to identify changes in tooth characteristics that are otherwise unobservable in a visual-tactile examination **Disadvantages:** uncertainty of the reliability of devices and the ability to detect disease and health
Electrical conductance	The demineralisation of the tooth is reported to	An adjunct to the visual examination	**Advantages:** the potential to identify changes in tooth characteristics

	have an effect on the tooth's electrical conductance. This is measured by placing a probe on the tooth which measures any potentially higher conductivity which occurs due to carious lesions being filled with saliva (Tam 2001)	203	that are otherwise unobservable in a visual-tactile examination **Disadvantages:** uncertainty of the reliability of devices and the ability to detect disease and health. Particularly due to the necessity to place the probe in an identical location for a reproducible result

References

1. Shafer WG. Textbook of Oral Pathology . 6th edition . Banglore : Prism book . Pvt. Ltd; 1997.p 405-452

2. Srilatha A,Doshi D, Kulkarni S,Reddy MP,Bharthi V.Advanced diagnostic aids in dental caries -A REVIEW .global oral health .2019; 2(2):118-27

3. Gomez J. Detection and diagnosis of the early caries lesion. BMC Oral Health. 2015;15 Suppl 1(Suppl 1):S3.

4. Colak H, Dülgergil CT, Dalli M, Hamidi MM. Early childhood caries update: A review of causes, diagnoses, and treatments. J Nat Sci Biol Med. 2013;4(1):29-38.

5. Macey R, Walsh T, Riley P, *et al.* Tests to detect and inform the diagnosis of caries. Cochrane Database Syst Rev. 2018;2018(12):CD013215.

6. Mohanraj M, Prabhu V,Senthil R.Diagnostic methods for early detection of dental caries -A Review. Int Pedod Rehabil.2016;1:29-36

7. Diamanti I, Berdouses ED, Kavvadia K, Arapostathis KN, Reppa C, Sifakaki M, Panagopoulou O, Polychronopoulou A, Oulis CJ. Caries prevalence and caries experience (ICDAS II criteria) of 5-, 12- and 15-year-old Greek children in relation to socio-demographic risk indicators. Trends at the national level in a period of a decade. Eur Arch Paediatr Dent. 2021;22(4):619-631

8. Tinanoff N, Baez RJ, Guillory CD, Donly KJ ,et al Early childhood caries epidemiology, aetiology, risk assessment, societal burden, management, education, and policy: Global perspective . Int J Paediatr Dent. 2019;29:238–248.

9. Cabral RN, Hilgert LA, Faber J, Leal SC. Caries risk assessment in schoolchildren--a form based on Cariogram software. J Appl Oral Sci. 2014 ;22(5):397-402.

10. Rathee M, Sapra A. Dental Caries. In: StatPearls [Internet]. Treasure Island (FL): StatPearls Publishing; 2021

11. Diagnosis and Management of Dental Caries Annika Julihn, Margaret Grindefjord, and Ivar Espelid

12. R G, Gopakumar M. Diagnostic Aids in Pediatric Dentistry. Int J Clin Pediatr Dent. 2011;4(1):1-7.

13. Dikmen B. Icdas II criteria (international caries detection and assessment system). J Istanb Univ Fac Dent. 2015 . 21;49(3):63-72.

14. Gugnani N, Pandit IK, Srivastava N, Gupta M, Sharma M. International Caries Detection and Assessment System (ICDAS): A New Concept. Int J Clin Pediatr Dent. 2011;4(2):93-100.

15. Shivakumar K, Prasad S, Chandu G. International Caries Detection and Assessment System: A new paradigm in detection of dental caries. J Conserv Dent. 2009;12(1):10-6.

16. Pitts NB, Ekstrand KR; ICDAS Foundation. International Caries Detection and Assessment System (ICDAS) and its International Caries Classification and Management System (ICCMS) - methods for staging of the caries process and enabling dentists to manage caries. Community Dent Oral Epidemiol. 2013;41(1):e41-52.

17. Mohanraj M, Prabhu VR, Senthil R. Diagnostic methods for early detedtion of dental caries – A review Int J Pedod Rehabil.2016;1:29-36

18. Shoaib L, Deery C, Ricketts DN, Nugent ZJ. Validity and reproducibility of ICDAS II in primary teeth. Caries Res. 2009;43(6):442-8.

19. Kühnisch J, Berger S, Goddon I, Senkel H, Pitts N, Heinrich-Weltzien R. Occlusal caries detection in permanent molars according to WHO basic methods, ICDAS II and laser fluorescence measurements. Community Dent Oral Epidemiol. 2008;36(6):475-84.

20. Rodrigues JA, Hug I, Diniz MB, Lussi A. Performance of fluorescence methods, radiographic examination and ICDAS II on occlusal surfaces in vitro. Caries Res. 2008;42(4):297-304.

21. Tassoker M, Ozcan S, Karabekiroglu S. Occlusal Caries Detection and Diagnosis Using Visual ICDAS Criteria, Laser Fluorescence Measurements, and Near-Infrared Light Transillumination Images. Med Princ Pract. 2020;29(1):25-31.

22. Laputková G, Schwartzová V, Bánovčin J, Alexovič M, Sabo J. Salivary Protein Roles in Oral Health and as Predictors of Caries Risk. Open Life Sci. 2018 18;13:174-200.

23. Abesi F, Mirshekar A, Moudi E, Seyedmajidi M, Haghanifar S, Haghighat N, *et al.* Diagnostic accuracy of digital and conventional radiography in the detection of non- cavitated approximal dental caries. Iran J Radiol 2012;9:17-21.

24. El-Samarrai S, Misbah MM. Diagnosis of initial carious lesion by clinical and conventional radiographic methods in comparison to direct digital radiography. J Baghdad Coll Dent 2007;19:77-80.

25. Pontual AA, de Melo DP, de Almeida SM, Bóscolo FN, Haiter Neto F. Comparison of digital systems and conventional dental film for the detection of approximal enamel caries. Dentomaxillofac Radiol 2010;39:431-6.

26. Gakenheimer DC. The efficacy of a computerized caries detector in intraoral digital radiography. J Am Dent Assoc. 2002 ;133(7):883-90.

27. Yilmaz and Keles . Recent Methods for diagnosis of Dental Caries in Dentistry. Meandros Med Dent J. 2018; 19:1-8

28. Valizadeh S, Ehsani S, Esmaeili F, Tavakoli MA. Accuracy of digital subtraction radiography in combination with a contrast media in assessment of proximal caries depth. J Dent Res Dent Clin Dent Prospects. 2008 ;2(3):77-8

29. Park JH, Choi YS, Hwang EH, Lee GJ, Choi S, Park YH, *et al.* Proximal caries detection using digital subtraction radiography in the artificial caries activity model. Korean J Oral Maxillofac Radiol 2009;39:35-9.

30. Paymani A, Talayeepour A, Anaraki SN, Mehralizadeh S, Delavar AS, Talebi S. Evaluation of the accuracy of digital subtraction radiography in the diagnosis of different depths of class III caries (An in vitro study). J Res Dent Sci 2011;8:120-9.

31. Shah N, Bansal N, Logani A. Recent advances in imaging technologies in dentistry. World J Radiol. 2014 28;6(10):794-807.

32. van Daatselaar AN, Tyndall DA, van der Stelt PF. Detection of caries with local CT. Dentomaxillofac Radiol. 2003;32(4):235-41

33. De Felice F, Di Carlo G, Saccucci M, Tombolini V, Polimeni A. Dental Cone Beam Computed Tomography in Children: Clinical Effectiveness and Cancer Risk due to Radiation Exposure. Oncology. 2019;96(4):173-178.

34. Valizadeh S, Tavakkoli MA, Karimi Vasigh H, Azizi Z, Zarrabian T. Evaluation of Cone Beam Computed Tomography (CBCT) System: Comparison with Intraoral Periapical Radiography in Proximal Caries Detection. J Dent Res Dent Clin Dent Prospects. 2012;6(1):1-5.

35. Hall AF, DeSchepper E, Ando M, Stookey GK. In vitro studies of laser fluorescence for detection and quantification of mineral loss from dental caries. Adv Dent Res. 1997;11:507-14.

36. Lo EC, Zhi QH, Itthagarun A. Comparing two quantitative methods for studying remineralization of artificial caries. J Dent. 2010;38:352-9.

37. Ie YL, Verdonschot EH. Performance of diagnostic systems in occlusal caries detection compared. Community Dent Oral Epidemiol. 1994;22(3):187-91.

38. Ismail AI. Clinical diagnosis of precavitated carious lesions. Community Dent Oral Epidemiol. 1997;25:13-23.

39. Peers A, Hill FJ, Mitropoulos CM, Holloway PJ. Validity and reproducibility of clinical examination, fibre-optic transillumination, and bite-wing radiology for the diagnosis of small approximal carious lesions: An in vitro study. Caries Res. 1993;27:307-11.

40. Vaarkamp J, ten Bosch J, Verdonschot EH, Huysmans MC. Wavelength-dependent fibre-optic transillumination of small

approximal caries lesions: the use of a dye, and a comparison to bitewing radiography. Caries Res. 1997;31(3):232-7.

41. Schneiderman A, Elbaum M, Shultz T, Keem S, Greenebaum M, Driller J. Assessment of dental caries with Digital Imaging Fiber-Optic TransIllumination (DIFOTI): in vitro study. Caries Res. 1997;31(2):103-10.

42. Bin-Shuwaish M, Yaman P, Dennison J, Neiva G. The correlation of DIFOTI to clinical and radiographic images in Class II carious lesions. J Am Dent Assoc. 2008 ;139(10):1374-81.

43. Krause F, Melner DJ, Stawirej R, Jepsen S, & Braun A(2008) LED based occlusal and approximal caries detec-tion in vitroJournal of Dental Research87(SpecialIssue B)Abstract 0526. [accessed Jan 07 2022].

44. Longbottom C, Huysmans MC. Electrical measurements for use in caries clinical trials. J Dent Res. 2004;83:C76-9.

45. Nokhbatolfoghahaie H, Alikhasi M, Chiniforush N, Khoei F, Safavi N, Yaghoub Zadeh B. Evaluation of Accuracy of DIAGNOdent in Diagnosis of Primary and Secondary Caries in Comparison to Conventional Methods. J Lasers Med Sci. 2013;4(4):159-167.

46. Bader JD, Shugars DA, Bonito AJ. Systematic reviews of selected dental caries diagnostic and management methods. J Dent Educ. 2001;65:960-8.

47. Hosoya Y, Taguchi T, Tay FR. Evaluation of a new caries detecting dye for primary and permanent carious dentin. J Dent. 2007 ;35(2):137-43

48. Yin W, Hu DY, Fan X, Feng Y, Zhang YP, Cummins D, Mateo LR, Pretty IA, Ellwood RP. A clinical investigation using quantitative light-induced fluorescence (QLF) of the anticaries efficacy of a dentifrice containing 1.5% arginine and 1450 ppm fluoride as sodium monofluorophosphate. J Clin Dent. 2013;24 Spec no A:A15-22.

49. Gimenez T, Braga MM, Raggio DP, Deery C, Ricketts DN, Mendes FM. Fluorescence-based methods for detecting caries lesions:

systematic review, meta-analysis and sources of heterogeneity. PLoS One. 2013 4;8(4):e60421

50. Stookey GK. Quantitative light fluorescence: a technology for early monitoring of the caries process. Dent Clin North Am. 2005 ;49(4):753-70

51. Ferreira Zandoná A, Santiago E, Eckert G, Fontana M, Ando M, Zero DT. Use of ICDAS combined with quantitative light-induced fluorescence as a caries detection method. Caries Res. 2010;44(3):317-22.

52. Heinrich-Weltzien R, Kühnisch J, Ifland S, Tranaeus S, Angmar-Månsson B, Stösser L. Detection of initial caries lesions on smooth surfaces by quantitative light-induced fluorescence and visual examination: an in vivo comparison. Eur J Oral Sci. 2005 ;113(6):494-8

53. Unlu N, Ermis RB, Sener S, Kucukyilmaz E, Cetin AR. An in vitro comparison of different diagnostic methods in detection of residual dentinal caries. Int J Dent. 2010;2010:864935.

54. Gimenez T, Braga MM, Raggio DP, Deery C, Ricketts DN, Mendes FM. Fluorescence-based methods for detecting caries lesions: systematic review, meta-analysis and sources of heterogeneity. PLoS One. 2013 4;8(4):e60421.

55. Guo L, Shi W. Salivary biomarkers for caries risk assessment. J Calif Dent Assoc. 2013 Feb;41(2):107-9, 112-8.

56. Laputková G, Schwartzová V, Bánovčin J, Alexovič M, Sabo J. Salivary Protein Roles in Oral Health and as Predictors of Caries Risk. Open Life Sci. 2018 18;13:174-200.

57. Abrams SH, Sivagurunathan KS, Silvertown JD, Wong B, Hellen A, Mandelis A, Hellen WMP, Elman GI, Mathew SM, Mensinkai PK, Amaechi BT. Correlation with Caries Lesion Depth of The Canary System, DIAGNOdent and ICDAS II. Open Dent J. 2017 29;11:679-689

58. KS, Silvertown JD, Wong B, Hellen A, Mandelis A, Hellen WMP, Elman GI, Mathew SM, Mensinkai PK, Amaechi BT. Correlation with

Caries Lesion Depth of The Canary System, DIAGNOdent and ICDAS II. Open Dent J. 2017 29;11:679-689.

59. Markowitz K, Gutta A, Merdad HE, Guzy G, Rosivack G. In vitro study of the diagnostic performance of the Spectra Caries Detection Aid. J Clin Dent. 2015;26(1):17-22

60. Xiao J, Luo J, Ly-Mapes O, Wu TT, Dye T,Al Jallad N, Hao P, Ruan J, Bullock S,Fiscella K .Assessing a Smartphone App (AICaries) That Uses Artificial Intelligence to Detect Dental Caries in Children and Provides Interactive Oral Health Education: Protocol for a Design and Usability Testing Study .JMIR Res Protoc 2021;10(10):e32921

61. Zhang X, Liang Y, Li W, Liu C, Gu D, Sun W, Miao L. Development and evaluation of deep learning for screening dental caries from oral photographs. Oral Dis. 2022 ;28(1):173-181

62. Lee JH, Kim DH, Jeong SN, Choi SH. Detection and diagnosis of dental caries using a deep learning-based convolutional neural network algorithm. J Dent. 2018 ;77:106-111.

63. Sharma V, Gupta N, Srivastava N, Rana V, Chandna P, Yadav S, Sharma A. Diagnostic potential of inflammatory biomarkers in early childhood caries - A case control study. Clin Chim Acta. 2017 ;471:158-163.

64. Børsting T, Venkatraman V, Fagerhaug TN, Skeie MS, Stafne SN, Feuerherm AJ, Sen A. Systematic assessment of salivary inflammatory markers and dental caries in children: an exploratory study. Acta Odontol Scand. 2021 7:1-8.

65. Ley B, Newton CA, Arnould I, Elicker BM, Henry TS, Vittinghoff E, Golden JA, Jones KD, Batra K, Torrealba J, Garcia CK, Wolters PJ. The MUC5B promoter polymorphism and telomere length in patients with chronic hypersensitivity pneumonitis: an observational cohort-control study. Lancet Respir Med. 2017 ;5(8):639-647

66. Reddy KV,Kumar KN, Subramaniyam V, Togani H,Kannaiah S,Reddy R

Dermatoglyphics:A new diagnostic tool in the detection of dental caries in children with special healthcare needs .Int J Pedod Rehabil 2018 ;3:18-22

67. Popovici D, Crauciuc E, Socolov R, Balan R, Hurjui L, Scripcariu I, Pavaleanu I. Early Diagnosis and Treatment of Dental Caries in Pregnancy. Maedica (Bucur). 2018 Jun;13(2):101-104..

68. Bhasin, Sudha, Anegundi R. Chairside simple caries activity test: Ora test .J Indian Soc Pedod Prev Dent.2006;24:76-9

69. Lee HS, Lee ES, Kang SM, Lee JH, Choi HJ, Kim BI. Clinical Assessment of a New Caries Activity Test Using Dental Plaque Acidogenicity in Children under Three Years of Age. J Clin Pediatr Dent. 2016;40(5):388-92.

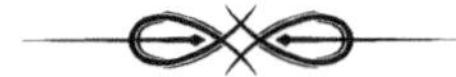